THE
PALEO DIET
MADE EASY

THE
PALEO
DIET
MADE EASY

LOVED BY
CELEBRITIES
& ATHLETES
ALIKE

EAT
LIKE YOUR
ANCESTORS TO
LOSE WEIGHT
& GET FIT

SIMPLE INGREDIENTS
NO JUNK → NO STARVING

OVER 100
RECIPES

JOY SKIPPER

hamlyn

An Hachette UK Company
www.hachette.co.uk

First published in Great Britain in 2014 by
Hamlyn, a division of Octopus Publishing Group Ltd
Endeavour House, 189 Shaftesbury Avenue, London, WC2H 8JY
www.octopusbooks.co.uk

ISBN 978-0-600-62932-0

A CIP catalogue record for this book is available from the British Library

Printed and bound by CPI Group (UK) Ltd, Croydon, CR0 4YY

10 9 8 7 6 5 4 3 2 1

Commissioning Editor: Eleanor Maxfield
Managing Editor: Clare Churly
Designer: Eoghan O'Brien
Design: Jeremy Tilston
Production Controller: Allison Gonsalves

NOTES:
Both metric and imperial measurements are given for the recipes. Use one
set of measures only, not a mixture of both.

Standard level spoon measurements are used in all recipes
1 tablespoon = 15 ml
1 teaspoon = 5 ml

Ovens should be preheated to the specified temperature. If using a fan-
assisted oven, follow the manufacturer's instructions for adjusting the time
and temperature. Grills should also be preheated.

This book includes dishes made with nuts and nut derivatives. It is advisable
for those with known allergic reactions to nuts and nut derivatives and those
who may be potentially vulnerable to these allergies, such as pregnant and
nursing mothers, invalids, the elderly, babies and children, to avoid dishes
made with nuts and nut oils.

The Department of Health advises that eggs should not be consumed raw.
This book contains some dishes made with raw or lightly cooked eggs. It is
prudent for more vulnerable people such as pregnant and nursing mothers,
invalids, the elderly, babies and young children to avoid uncooked or lightly
cooked dishes made with eggs.

CONTENTS

THE PALEO DIET

INTRODUCTION

This book will introduce you to the concept of the diet believed
to have been eaten by our ancestors thousands of years ago,
enabling them to stay lean and healthy. The book explains the basics
of the diet, plus gives lots of tips and ideas to help you get started,
and includes more than a hundred recipes to incorporate into your
everyday life.

The Paleolithic diet (known as the Paleo diet) is often referred
to as the hunter-gatherer diet and includes any food that could
be hunted or found, such as meats, fish, nuts, leafy greens and seeds.
It is based on the concept that the best diet is the one to which
we are genetically adapted, with the premise that human genetics
have hardly changed since the dawn of agriculture, and on research
showing that the aged populations of hunter-gatherer societies were
virtually free of high cholesterol, diabetes, obesity, hypertension
and other chronic diseases that have become endemic in Western
societies. There are signs that indicate our modern diet full of refined
foods, trans fats and sugar is the root of most degenerative diseases,
including cancer and heart disease, depression and fertility problems.
We have changed our diets, but our genetics have not changed
enough to accommodate them.

Over the past couple of years a number of authors have written about
the Paleo diet, each with their own variation. It's very difficult for us
to know for certain what Paleo people ate or how they lived, but in
essence the Paleo diet is based around a much more nutrient-dense,
toxin-free, whole-food diet than that which is currently being eaten
today. The best way to think of this diet is as a particular approach to
eating, with a template that can be adjusted to suit each individual's
biochemical needs. It is also important to think of it not so much as
a diet, but as a healthy eating regime that can be maintained for life.

HOW TO USE THE BOOK

The great thing about the Paleo diet is that once you know what you
can and cannot eat, there is nothing else to worry about! No calorie
counting, no weighing of foods – the foods you are allowed can be

eaten as often as you wish. The only foods that need to be limited are root vegetables and fruit (see page 17), as these are high in starch and sugar, and if excess sugar is not burned off it will turn to fat.

This book provides you with recipes featuring only the allowed foods, and these can be used to make meals and snacks throughout the day. The recipes will give you ideas of ways to use the many foods available on the Paleo diet – as long as you stick to those foods, you can also experiment with your own recipes, too.

So what can you eat? Anything that the hunter-gatherer would have been able to forage for – meats (Paleolithic man would have found wild meat, so the leanest cuts you can find are best), fish and seafood, vegetables, fruits, eggs, nuts and seeds. You may also reduce your toxin intake by choosing nutrient-dense organic foods. Foods to avoid include all grains, legumes and pulses, dairy and refined sugars (see page 12).

The Paleo diet is a diet that can be followed for life, not just as a short-term weight-loss regime. It is a healthy, long-term eating regime that has been shown to reduce a number of modern diseases.

IS THE PALEO DIET FOR EVERYONE?

There is no such thing as an optimal diet for the whole world – think of the diet of the Inuit or Masai who eat high-fat diets, yet remain healthy. So it's important to remember that our ancestors didn't all eat the same diet – there was a wide variation in the proportion of protein, carbohydrate and fat consumed, and the different types of food consumed by different populations around the world.

We are all individual, with individual lifestyles, and we grew up in different environments, with different toxin exposure and different experiences, so many of our genes are the same, but some are different, and the way some of them may have been expressed may also be different. So the Paleo diet is about finding a diet that works for you.

If you have been on a diet that was based on a lot of processed food for many years, along with high alcohol and toxin intake, the transition to a nutrient-dense, low-toxic diet may not be a smooth one. This doesn't mean that the Paleo diet is not for you, it may just mean you have some work to do on your digestive system or other systems in the body, to ensure that you are digesting and detoxifying optimally first. There is no such thing as a quick fix, especially if you have been on a heavily processed food diet for a long time.

Two groups of people that may struggle with this diet are vegetarians and vegans as, being based on a hunter-gatherer diet, it includes meat, poultry, fish and eggs. And without legumes and grains, vegetarians and vegans will not be able to sustain a balanced diet with sufficient protein intake.

HOW DOES THE DIET WORK?

A Paleo diet is naturally lower in carbohydrate than the modern diet and automatically eliminates many foods that are low in nutrients and high in calories. It will also eliminate processed foods that are high in hidden sugars, fats and toxins, and reduce the intake of foods that may cause intolerances or allergies, or foods that may be hard to digest. The carbohydrates on the Paleo diet (fruit and vegetables) are also low glycaemic index, meaning that they cause slow and limited rises in your blood sugar and insulin levels. Your body's blood sugar balance may be improved, as you will be eating more protein and good fat that will sustain your appetite for longer.

HEALTH BENEFITS

There are a number of reasons why this diet is healthy, some of which have already been mentioned, including cutting out toxins and increasing your intake of nutrient-dense foods.

When you consider that the body is made up of protein, carbohydrates and fats, it makes sense that if you feed your body those nutrients in the cleanest form possible then it will perform better.

By eliminating processed foods you are automatically eating a low-sodium diet while increasing your intake of potassium (rich in many vegetables, nuts and seeds), and the combination of low sodium and high potassium is a recipe for good vascular health and low blood pressure.

Clinical trials have shown that the Paleo diet may lower the risk of cardiovascular disease, blood pressure and markers of inflammation, help with weight loss, reduce acne and promote optimum health and athletic performance.

THE PALEO DIET AND EXERCISE

As with all healthy eating plans, you will see better results if you are active. Hunter-gatherers were physically active on a daily basis, while they were seeking food, water and shelter. We no longer have to do these things, but taking regular exercise may be beneficial, both for weight loss and long-term health.

If you are intending to follow the Paleo diet and have not been taking regular exercise, seek help from a professional to be assessed for the level of exercise you should start with.

If you are a training athlete you will no doubt be wondering if this diet will suit you. Not so long ago, carbohydrates were the endurance nutrient of choice, and protein was the focus of all body builders and strength athletes, but things have moved on since then. The Paleo diet is naturally high in animal protein, which is the richest source of branched-chain amino acids, needed for building and repairing muscles. It also reduces muscle loss as the diet is very alkaline (one way the body neutralizes an acid-producing diet is by breaking down muscle). The high intake of vegetables and fruit also ensures a high intake of vitamins, minerals and phytochemicals, which help to support the immune system, an important issue for all athletes.

WHAT TO EXPECT ON THE DIET

If your present diet is high in processed foods, coffee, alcohol, wheat and dairy, it may take you a while to adjust to your new diet and to find the foods that work for you. Keeping a food diary from day one may be helpful with this, as it's hard to remember how you felt and if any foods affected you in any way.

You may also get withdrawal symptoms from cutting out some of the old foods so it could be a while before you start to feel better and see your body shape change.

GETTING STARTED

If you find the thought of a 'diet' a bit daunting, set yourself a time challenge to start with. Commit to a 30-day period where you eliminate the foods suggested below, therefore reducing toxins and food sensitivities, and so reducing allergic reactions, and introduce the new foods that may have been absent from your diet, which may hopefully improve digestion, boost energy, regulate sugar balance and normalize weight. Once you start to get to grips with your new eating regime you may find some foods agree with you more than others, so you can start to tailor the diet to suit your individual needs.

Here is a basic list of foods to eat and not eat:

Eat:
- Grass-produced meats (grain causes the same problem in animals as it does in humans)
- Fish (wild is best, to avoid mercury and other toxins found in farmed fish)
- Seafood
- Fresh fruit (limit the amount if you are trying to lose weight as it is high in natural sugar)
- Fresh vegetables
- Eggs (look for omega-3 enriched)
- Nuts
- Seeds
- Healthy oil – olive, flaxseed, avocado, coconut, walnut

Don't eat:
- Legumes (including peanuts) and pulses
- Dairy
- Cereal grains
- Refined sugar
- Potatoes
- Processed foods
- Salt

TOP TIPS FOR BEGINNERS

Sticking to a new eating regime can be difficult when there are outside influences, such as work or family, to juggle, too, so the following tips may be useful:

- **Set small, achievable targets** – try including a new food each week or increasing your exercise by walking to a further bus-stop each morning.

- **Get support** – get your family or friends involved by asking them to join you on the diet. That way, if you are cooking for the whole family you won't have to make separate meals, and everyone will benefit!

- **Don't get hungry** – ensure that you plan your day with sufficient healthy snacks that mean you never get hungry; eating little and often is fine as long as it is based on the foods you are allowed. Maintain your appetite throughout the day, which will also help to keep your blood sugar balanced, causing less stress on the body. The less hungry you are, the easier it is to lose weight!

- **Be aware of what you are eating** – don't fall into the trap of 'mindless eating', just eating because food is there or has been offered. Eat in a conscious way, and savour each mouthful.

- **Personalize the diet to suit you** – it may take a few weeks for you to get to know which foods you like and which suit you. You also have your own routine and it's important to make your diet work around that.

- **Make changes that are sustainable** – gradually change your diet to suit you and make sure the changes you make are those that can be maintained for life, not just for a few weeks.

10 WAYS TO MAKE THE PALEO DIET WORK FOR YOU

①

BE ORGANIZED

Spend time at the beginning of the week to shop and prepare food for the week ahead.

②

PLAN AHEAD

Plan your meals in advance so you have something tasty to look forward to, so that you don't get hungry and reach for the wrong foods.

③

TAKE FOODS WITH YOU

If you work away from home, make yourself delicious lunches to take with you.

④

RESTOCK THE CUPBOARDS AND FRIDGE

Only have Paleo foods in the house; that way, you will never be tempted to cheat!

⑤

VEGGIE BOX DELIVERY

Sign up to a veggie box delivery scheme to ensure you are eating fresh organic vegetables each week. You may even get to try some new ones you didn't know you liked.

⑥ KEEP IT SIMPLE

With each meal or snack, first include protein (meat, poultry, fish or eggs), then add some vegetables or fruit.

⑦ EAT REGULARLY

Don't let yourself get hungry. Eat little and often; having snacks, such as a small handful of nuts and seeds with a piece of fruit, will sustain you between meals.

⑧ EAT A RAINBOW!

Vegetables are loaded with essential vitamins, minerals, enzymes, antioxidants, fibre and water, all essential for optimum health. The colour of your fruit and vegetables is linked to the nutrients they include, so eat as many colourful fruit and veg a day as you can – variety is key.

⑨ USE THE 80:20 RULE

If you find you have a day or night when you really cannot stick to the diet (for example, you are invited out to dinner), don't worry, just count it as your 20% of being non-Paleo for that week, and get right back on to the Paleo eating regime the next day.

⑩ START A FOOD DIARY

Keep a note of what you eat, how you feel and how you sleep. Hopefully over time you will see positive changes and may be able to relate them to foods you are consuming.

FREQUENTLY ASKED QUESTIONS

Can a vegetarian or vegan follow the Paleo diet?
As the Paleo diet is based on what a hunter-gatherer would have caught/found, it naturally includes meat. It is important to include protein in the diet, which most vegetarians or vegans would gain from eating legumes, cereals and pulses, but these foods contain anti-nutrients that may have a negative effect (see below).

Is it suitable for children?
If you can get your child to eat enough vegetables, this diet is fine for children – they really don't need all the refined carbohydrates (pizza, pasta etc.) to enable them to grow, as they can get carbohydrates (along with fibre, vitamins and minerals) from vegetables.

Is it suitable during pregnancy?
As the diet is rich in fresh fruit, vegetables, organic meat and fish it is fine for pregnancy.

How will I get my intake of calcium for my bones without dairy?
Bone health is mainly dependent on an acid/alkaline dietary balance. If the acid in the body is too high, then calcium is 'pulled' from the bones to neutralize it. Acid-producing foods include cheese, grains, legumes and salted foods, whereas fruit and vegetables are alkaline, so increasing these in your diet should bring the acid/alkaline, and therefore the calcium, back into balance. Leafy green vegetables, such as kale, and some nuts (almonds) and seeds (sesame) are also rich in calcium.

Is organic food really better for you?
There is always lots of debate about this, but research has shown that foods that have had to battle the elements to survive and grow without the help of pesticides and fertilizers are likely to be more nutrient-dense than those that had help.

Will I lose weight on the Paleo diet?

If your present diet has been high in processed foods and refined carbohydrates there is a good chance that you may lose weight, as you will be eating foods that are easier for the body to recognize and digest.

How much fruit can I eat on the diet?

In general, fresh fruits are healthy foods that are good sources of minerals, vitamins and fibre. However, the fruits we eat today are sweeter, larger and contain less fibre than their wild counterparts, so if you are trying to lose weight it may be beneficial to limit high-sugar fruits, such as bananas, mangoes, grapes, apples, pineapples and kiwi fruits, and try to include more vegetables in your diet instead. Root vegetables, however, are higher in starch and sugar than leafy green vegetables, and so should be eaten in moderation, too.

Why no beans?

Beans contain lectins, which are carbohydrate-binding proteins present in most plants, especially seeds, beans and tubers like cereals, potatoes and beans. Until recently, their main use was as histology and blood transfusion reagents, but in the past two decades it has been realized that many lectins are toxic and inflammatory.

Which oils are allowed on the Paleo diet?

There are many different views on the kinds of oils that should be consumed when following the Paleo diet. The consensus, however, seems to be that oils from all the plants that are allowed can be consumed: olive oil (great for salads and sautéing, but don't heat too high); coconut oil (high in saturated fats but withstands high cooking temperatures so good for stir-fries); avocado oil (delicious in salad dressings or cooking at low temperatures); and sesame oil (very rich in flavour, so only a small amount is needed and it is not recommended as an everyday oil). Oils that should not be used are those rich in omega-6 fatty acids, plus oils from legumes, soy etc. (groundnut oil, vegetable oil, sunflower oil, corn oil, rapeseed oil).

What can I drink and use instead of milk?
Almond milk and coconut milk.

Can I eat peanuts on the Paleo diet?
No, they are legumes.

Is alcohol allowed on the diet?
Alcohol is not allowed on the diet, although if you occasionally add wine to food when you are cooking, just be sure to burn off the alcohol.

Is the Paleo diet expensive?
The diet does not have to be expensive, especially if you normally buy pre-prepared food – cooking from scratch is not only healthier, but cheaper, too. Shop around to get the best prices, buy from local markets, and maybe even think about growing your own organic vegetables!

Can I get most of the ingredients at a supermarket?
Yes, all Paleo foods are readily available in supermarkets, including the fresh ingredients. If you have a good butcher and fishmonger nearby, you may also want to visit them to see what offers they have and get advice about cooking the best joints of meat or fresh fish.

Any tips for what to grab on the run?
Nuts, seeds and fruit are the easiest foods to carry around.

1

BREAKFASTS

SMOKED HADDOCK SCRAMBLED EGGS

This protein-rich breakfast sets you up for a busy day.

SERVES 2
PREPARATION TIME 10 MINUTES
COOKING TIME 12 MINUTES

1 bay leaf
1 thyme sprig
1 garlic clove
4 whole peppercorns
150 ml (¼ pint) non-dairy milk
100 g (3½ oz) smoked haddock fillet
4 large eggs, beaten
2 tablespoons chopped chives
freshly ground black pepper

1 Place the bay leaf, thyme, garlic, peppercorns and milk in a pan and slowly bring to a simmer. Add the smoked haddock, turn off the heat and leave to stand for 6 minutes.

2 Remove the haddock from the poaching liquid and flake into large pieces, discarding the skin and any bones. Reserve 2 tablespoons of the poaching liquid.

3 Heat a nonstick saucepan over a low heat, add the eggs and cook for a few minutes, stirring occasionally, until just scrambled, then add the haddock and reserved poaching liquid and cook for a further minute.

4 Stir in the chives, season with pepper and serve immediately.

CHORIZO AND EGG-TOPPED BAKED MUSHROOMS

Chorizo has a very distinct taste and the mushrooms bring out the best of its flavour.

SERVES 2
PREPARATION TIME 10 MINUTES
COOKING TIME 15–17 MINUTES

2 large Portobello mushrooms, cleaned, stalks removed and chopped
1 tablespoon olive oil
25 g (1 oz) chorizo sausage, sliced
2 spring onions, sliced
100 g (3½ oz) small button mushrooms, sliced
1 tablespoon chopped parsley
2 eggs
freshly ground black pepper

1 Place the Portobello mushrooms on a baking sheet, gill sides up, and drizzle with half the oil. Bake in a preheated oven, 200°C (400°F), Gas Mark 6, for 15 minutes.

2 Meanwhile, heat the remaining oil in a frying pan, add the chorizo and cook for 3–4 minutes. Add the spring onions and cook for a further 2–3 minutes until softened. Add the sliced button mushrooms and chopped stalks and continue to cook for 8–10 minutes. Stir in half the parsley.

3 Towards the end of the cooking time, poach the eggs in a separate small saucepan of simmering water for 3–5 minutes, or until cooked to your liking.

4 Divide the chorizo mixture between the Portobello mushrooms and top each one with a poached egg.

5 Season with pepper, sprinkle over the remaining parsley and serve.

HUEVOS RANCHEROS

A traditional Mexican farming dish, this is a delicious way to serve eggs in the morning. If you want a little more spice, just add a finely diced red chilli to the pepper mixture, too.

SERVES 4
PREPARATION TIME 10 MINUTES
COOKING TIME 15 MINUTES

3 tablespoons olive oil
1 large onion, diced
2 red peppers, cored, deseeded
   and diced
2 garlic cloves, crushed
¾ teaspoon dried oregano
2 x 400 g (13 oz) cans chopped
   tomatoes
4 eggs
pinch of smoked paprika
1 tablespoon chopped parsley,
   to garnish

1 Heat 2 tablespoons of the oil in a frying pan, add the onion, red peppers, garlic and oregano and sauté for 5 minutes until softened.

2 Add the tomatoes and cook for a further 5 minutes, then pour into a shallow ovenproof dish and keep warm.

3 Heat the remaining oil in a large clean frying pan, add the eggs and fry until the whites are set and the yolks are cooked to your liking.

4 Serve the eggs on top of the tomato sauce, sprinkled with the smoked paprika and parsley.

BREAKFAST TORTILLA

Tortillas are simple to make, and you can add any vegetables of your choice. Prepare in advance and serve in wedges for breakfast, or wrap them up for a perfect packed lunch.

SERVES 4
PREPARATION TIME 10 MINUTES
COOKING TIME 25–30 MINUTES

2 tablespoons olive oil
2 shallots, diced
4 bacon rashers, fat removed and chopped
250 g (8 oz) chestnut mushrooms, sliced
6 large eggs
150 g (5 oz) cherry tomatoes, halved
1 tablespoon chopped parsley
freshly ground black pepper

1 Heat 1 tablespoon of the oil in a frying pan with a flameproof handle, add the shallots and bacon and cook for 3–4 minutes until the shallots have softened. Add the mushrooms and cook for a further 5–6 minutes until soft. Remove the mixture with a slotted spoon and set aside.

2 Beat the eggs in a large bowl and season with pepper, then stir in the bacon mixture, tomatoes and parsley.

3 Heat the remaining oil in the frying pan over a high heat, pour in the egg mixture and cook for 1–2 minutes. Reduce the temperature to low and cook for a further 12–15 minutes, keeping an eye on the edges to make sure it is not overcooked underneath – the top should still be runny.

4 Place the pan under a preheated grill and cook the top until golden and bubbling. To turn out, place a plate on top of the tortilla and carefully turn the pan upside down. Serve the tortilla hot or cold, cut into wedges.

BAKED EGGS WITH SPINACH AND HAM

This is a great weekend breakfast treat! And if you want to spice it up, add a finely diced red chilli to the tomato mixture.

SERVES 2
PREPARATION TIME 10 MINUTES
COOKING TIME 25 MINUTES

1 tablespoon olive oil
1 onion, diced
1 garlic clove, crushed
400 g (13 oz) can chopped
    tomatoes
100 ml (3½ fl oz) water
100 g (3½ oz) roasted peppers,
    homemade or from a jar, sliced
175 g (6 oz) lean ham, shredded
50 g (2 oz) baby spinach leaves
2 eggs
pinch of smoked paprika
freshly ground black pepper

1 Heat the oil in an ovenproof frying pan, add the onion and cook for 4–5 minutes until softened. Add the garlic and cook for a further minute.

2 Pour in the tomatoes and measurement water and season with pepper, then stir in the roasted peppers and ham. Bring to a simmer and cook for 10 minutes.

3 Stir in the spinach and when it starts to wilt make 2 hollows in the sauce. Crack an egg into each hollow and sprinkle with a pinch of paprika.

4 Transfer to a preheated oven, 180°C (350°F), Gas Mark 4, for 10 minutes, or until the egg whites have set.

DIPPY EGG WITH ASPARAGUS SOLDIERS

Asparagus and eggs are a perfect combination, so why not try them for breakfast or brunch?

SERVES 1
PREPARATION TIME 5 MINUTES, PLUS COOLING
COOKING TIME 6–8 MINUTES

1 tablespoon hazelnuts
4–5 asparagus spears, woody ends snapped off
1 large egg

1 Heat a dry nonstick frying pan over a medium-low heat and dry-fry the hazelnuts for 3–4 minutes, shaking the pan occasionally, until golden brown and toasted. Leave to cool slightly, then chop and set aside.

2 Cook the asparagus in a large saucepan of boiling water for 3–4 minutes until just tender.

3 Meanwhile, in a separate small saucepan, boil the egg in boiling water for 3–4 minutes until soft-boiled.

4 Drain the asparagus, place on a warmed plate and sprinkle with the chopped hazelnuts.

5 Place the egg in an eggcup on the same plate and serve.

BREAKFAST BANANA SPLIT

Banana split usually includes ice cream, but this lovely breakfast will get you off to a healthy start instead!

SERVES 2
PREPARATION TIME 5 MINUTES
COOKING TIME 4–5 MINUTES

1 tablespoon coconut oil
1 tablespoon clear honey
2 bananas, halved lengthways
2 tablespoons flaked almonds
25 g (1 oz) walnuts
1 orange
1 dessert apple, grated

1 Heat the oil and honey in a frying pan until melted and sizzling. Add the bananas, cut side down, and cook for 3–4 minutes until golden.

2 Meanwhile, heat a separate dry nonstick frying pan over a medium-low heat and dry-fry the flaked almonds and walnuts for 3–4 minutes, shaking the pan occasionally, until golden brown and toasted.

3 Grate the rind of the orange into a bowl, then, using a sharp knife, remove the peel and pith from the orange. Cut out the segments and add to the bowl with the grated apple. Mix together.

4 Spoon the bananas on to 4 warmed plates and top with the apple and orange mixture. Sprinkle over the toasted nuts and serve drizzled with the juices from the pan.

2

SOUPS

SALMON AND HORSERADISH SOUP

The creaminess of the salmon and the heat of the horseradish go really well together in this soup.

SERVES 4
PREPARATION TIME 15 MINUTES
COOKING TIME 30 MINUTES

475 g (15 oz) cauliflower, broken into florets
1 tablespoon olive oil
1 onion, chopped
1 leek, trimmed, cleaned and shredded
275 g (9 oz) swede, peeled and diced
1.2 litres (2 pints) fish stock
2 tomatoes, chopped
500 g (1 lb) skinless salmon fillet, cut into large chunks
100 ml (3½ fl oz) non-dairy milk
1 teaspoon grated fresh horseradish
juice of ½ lemon
1 small bunch of dill, roughly chopped
freshly ground black pepper

1 Cook the cauliflower in a saucepan of boiling water for 4–5 minutes just until tender. Drain and set aside.

2 Meanwhile, heat the oil in a separate large saucepan, add the onion and leek and sauté for 3–4 minutes until softened. Add the swede and cook for a further 2 minutes.

3 Pour in the stock and bring to the boil, then reduce the heat, cover and simmer for 10 minutes. Add the tomatoes and drained cauliflower and cook for a further 4–5 minutes.

4 Gently stir in the salmon and cook for 5 minutes, or until just cooked through.

5 Stir in the milk, horseradish and lemon juice and bring to a simmer, then sprinkle in the dill and season with pepper. Ladle the soup into warmed bowls and serve.

SMOKED HADDOCK AND SWEETCORN CHOWDER

The chowder can also be made with smoked cod or even thick chunks of smoked salmon.

SERVES 4
PREPARATION TIME 10 MINUTES
COOKING TIME 10–12 MINUTES

1 tablespoon olive oil
1 onion, chopped
2 celery sticks, sliced
300 g (10 oz) frozen or canned sweetcorn
600 ml (1 pint) vegetable stock
600 ml (1 pint) non-dairy milk
375 g (12 oz) smoked haddock fillet, skinned and cut into bite-sized pieces
1 tablespoon chopped parsley, to garnish

1 Heat the oil in a saucepan, add the onion and celery and sauté for 4–5 minutes until softened. Add the sweetcorn and cook, stirring, for 2 minutes.

2 Pour in the stock and milk and bring to the boil, then add the fish and simmer for 4–5 minutes, or until the fish is cooked through.

3 Ladle the soup into warmed bowls and serve sprinkled with the parsley.

ROASTED TOMATO AND GARLIC SOUP

Roasting tomatoes before using them for soup brings out their natural sweetness.

SERVES 4
PREPARATION TIME 10 MINUTES
COOKING TIME 25 MINUTES

1 kg (2 lb) ripe tomatoes, halved
4 garlic cloves, unpeeled
2 tablespoons olive oil
1 onion, chopped
1 carrot, peeled and chopped
1 celery stick, sliced
1 red pepper, cored, deseeded
   and chopped
700 ml (1⅛ pints) hot vegetable
   stock
freshly ground black pepper

1 Place the tomato halves and garlic cloves in a roasting tin. Sprinkle with 1 tablespoon of the oil and season with pepper. Roast in a preheated oven, 200°C (400F), Gas Mark 6, for 20 minutes.

2 Halfway through the tomato cooking time, heat the remaining oil in a saucepan, add the onion, carrot, celery and red pepper and sauté over a low heat for 10 minutes until softened.

3 Remove the garlic cloves from the roasted tomatoes and squeeze the garlic flesh into the saucepan with the sautéed vegetables, then tip in the roasted tomatoes and all the juices, and stir in the stock.

4 Using a hand blender, blend the soup until smooth. Reheat to a simmer, then ladle the soup into warmed bowls and serve.

LEEK AND ROCKET SOUP

A simple and quick way to make soup, which works equally well with watercress if you don't have any rocket.

SERVES 4
PREPARATION TIME 5 MINUTES
COOKING TIME 14–18 MINUTES

1 tablespoon olive oil
500 g (1 lb) leeks, trimmed,
   cleaned and sliced
500 ml (17 fl oz) hot vegetable
   stock
60 g (2¼ oz) rocket leaves
200 ml (7 fl oz) non-dairy milk
freshly ground black pepper

1 Heat the oil in a saucepan, add the leeks and sauté for 8-10 minutes until softened.

2 Add the stock and rocket leaves. Simmer for 4-6 minutes, then add the milk.

3 Using a hand blender, blend the soup until smooth. Reheat to a simmer and season with pepper. Ladle the soup into warmed bowls and serve.

ONION SOUP

Traditional French onion soup takes a while to make, but it is worth the effort. Letting the onions caramelize slowly gives the soup an intense, sweet flavour.

SERVES 4
PREPARATION TIME 10 MINUTES
COOKING TIME 45–50 MINUTES

1 tablespoon olive oil
1 kg (2 lb) onions, thinly sliced
2 tablespoons thyme leaves
1.2 litres (2 pints) beef stock
freshly ground black pepper

1 Heat the oil in a saucepan, add the onions and thyme leaves and cook over a low heat for 18–20 minutes until the onions are soft. Increase the heat and cook for a further 15–18 minutes, stirring occasionally, until the onions darken and start to caramelize.

2 Pour in the stock and bring to the boil, then reduce the heat and simmer for 10 minutes. Season with pepper, then ladle the soup into warmed bowls and serve.

3 Alternatively, to let the flavour develop, the soup can be cooled, then stored in the refrigerator for 24 hours before reheating.

GAZPACHO

• •

Gazpacho is a wonderful summer soup, made when all the seasonal ingredients are at their best – use the ripest ingredients you can find.

• •

SERVES 4
PREPARATION TIME 15 MINUTES

4 spring onions, chopped
2 garlic cloves
1 red pepper, cored, deseeded
   and chopped
½ cucumber
1 kg (2 lb) ripe plum tomatoes,
   halved
juice of 1 lemon
3 tablespoons olive oil

TO SERVE
1 hard-boiled egg, shelled and
   chopped
1 avocado, stoned, peeled and
   chopped

1 Place the spring onions, garlic and red pepper in a food processor or blender and blitz until broken down. Add the cucumber, tomatoes and lemon juice and process again.

2 Add 2 tablespoons of the oil and blend to your preferred consistency (you can make this soup as smooth or chunky as liked).

3 Pour into 4 bowls, then top with the chopped egg and avocado and a drizzle of the remaining oil. Serve immediately.

CHILLED AVOCADO SOUP WITH RED PEPPER SALSA

This cold, creamy soup is ideal for a summer's day. And it is rich in essential fats, too.

SERVES 4
PREPARATION TIME 15 MINUTES,
  PLUS CHILLING
COOKING TIME 2–3 MINUTES

4 large avocados
juice of 1 lime
½ red chilli, deseeded and finely
  diced
900 ml (1½ pints) vegetable
  stock, chilled
freshly ground black pepper
ice cubes, to serve

FOR THE SALSA
2 tablespoons pumpkin seeds
2 spring onions, finely sliced
½ red pepper, cored, deseeded
  and diced
¼ cucumber, diced
1 tablespoon coriander leaves
2 tablespoons olive oil
2 teaspoons lemon juice

1 Halve, stone and peel the avocados, then roughly chop the flesh and place in a food processor or blender with the lime juice, chilli and stock. Blend until smooth, then season with pepper and chill for 15 minutes.

2 Meanwhile, heat a dry nonstick frying pan over a medium-low heat and dry-fry the pumpkin seeds for 2–3 minutes, shaking the pan occasionally, until golden brown and toasted. Leave to cool.

3 To make the salsa, place the toasted pumpkin seeds in a bowl, add the remaining ingredients and mix together.

4 Place a couple of ice cubes in each of 4 shallow bowls, then pour over the soup. Spoon over the salsa and serve immediately.

TOMATO, SAFFRON AND ALMOND SOUP

This unusual combination of ingredients makes a warming, tasty soup.

SERVES 4
PREPARATION TIME 5 MINUTES
COOKING TIME 35–40 MINUTES

1 tablespoon olive oil
1 onion, chopped
1 garlic clove, crushed
2 x 400 g (13 oz) cans chopped tomatoes
1 litre (1¾ pints) vegetable stock
big pinch of saffron threads
75 g (3 oz) ground almonds
freshly ground black pepper

1 Heat the oil in a saucepan, add the onion and garlic and cook for 4–5 minutes until softened.

2 Add the tomatoes, stock and saffron and bring to the boil, then reduce the heat and simmer for 25–30 minutes.

3 Stir in the ground almonds and season with pepper, then cook for a further 5 minutes until starting to thicken.

4 Using a hand blender, blend the soup until smooth. Reheat to a simmer, then ladle the soup into warmed bowls and serve.

3

SALADS

SPINACH AND SALMON SALAD WITH ROCKET PESTO

Pesto is usually made with basil leaves, but there is no reason why you can't use other leaves such as rocket or parsley.

SERVES 4
PREPARATION TIME 10 MINUTES
COOKING TIME 6–8 MINUTES

4 salmon fillets, about 150 g
  (5 oz) each
1 tablespoon extra-virgin olive oil
450 g (14½ oz) baby spinach leaves
25 g (1 oz) pine nuts
juice of 1 lemon

FOR THE PESTO
100 g (3½ oz) rocket leaves
1 garlic clove
25 g (1 oz) pine nuts
4 tablespoons extra-virgin olive oil

1 To make the pesto, place the rocket, garlic and pine nuts in a food processor or blender and blitz until broken down. With the motor still running, slowly add the oil through the feeder tube until it forms a loose paste. Set aside.

2 Cook the salmon under a preheated hot grill for 3–4 minutes on each side, until the fish is cooked through.

3 Meanwhile, heat the oil in a frying pan, add the spinach and cook until just lightly wilted. Turn off the heat.

4 Flake the salmon into large pieces, discarding the skin and any bones, and place in a large salad bowl. Add the spinach and rocket pesto and toss together. Sprinkle with the pine nuts and serve drizzled with the lemon juice.

SESAME SEARED TUNA WITH ORIENTAL SALAD

Tuna is a meaty fish, but do not overcook it as it will become tough. Make sure the pan is hot so you can cook the tuna very quickly.

SERVES 2
PREPARATION TIME 15 MINUTES, PLUS MARINATING AND RESTING
COOKING TIME 4–6 MINUTES

2 teaspoons clear honey
1 teaspoon sesame oil
4 cm (1½ inch) piece of fresh root ginger, grated
2 tuna steaks, about 150 g (5 oz) each
2–3 tablespoons sesame seeds
juice of 1 lime

FOR THE SALAD
½ cucumber, cut into matchsticks
3 carrots, peeled and cut into matchsticks
6 spring onions, shredded
small handful of coriander leaves

1 Whisk together the honey, oil and ginger in a small bowl. Place the tuna in a non-metallic bowl, pour over the marinade and leave to marinate at room temperature for 10 minutes, turning once.

2 Meanwhile, to make the salad, mix together all the ingredients in a bowl. Set aside.

3 Heat a griddle pan or frying pan until hot. Scatter the sesame seeds on a plate, then coat the tuna in the seeds.

4 Cook the tuna in the hot pan for 2–3 minutes on each side, or until browned but still pink in the centre. Leave to rest for 2 minutes.

5 Thinly slice the tuna and serve on the salad, drizzled with the lime juice.

CRAB AND AVOCADO SALAD

Creamy avocado, sweet crabmeat and crunchy pecans make this a delicious Paleo salad.

SERVES 2
PREPARATION TIME 10 MINUTES, PLUS COOLING
COOKING TIME 3–4 MINUTES

1 tablespoon pecan nuts
50 g (2 oz) baby spinach leaves
25 g (1 oz) watercress
1 avocado
50 g (2 oz) cherry tomatoes, halved
100 g (3½ oz) white crabmeat

FOR THE DRESSING
2 tablespoons olive oil
juice of 1 lime
½ teaspoon Dijon mustard
½ teaspoon clear honey
1 tablespoon chopped coriander

1 Heat a dry nonstick frying pan over a medium-low heat and dry-fry the pecans for 3–4 minutes, shaking the pan occasionally, until golden brown and toasted. Set aside.

2 To make the dressing, whisk together all the ingredients in a small bowl.

3 Divide the spinach leaves and watercress between 2 plates. Halve, stone and peel the avocado, then slice the flesh and divide between the plates.

4 Top with the remaining ingredients and drizzle with the dressing. Serve immediately.

PRAWN, WATERMELON AND AVOCADO SALAD

Enjoy this healthy, tasty salad in the summer. And if you have any leftover watermelon to use up, put it in a blender and blend to make a refreshing smoothie.

SERVES 4
PREPARATION TIME 10 MINUTES, PLUS STANDING

1 small red onion, finely sliced
1 garlic clove, crushed
1 red chilli, deseeded and finely diced
juice of 1 lime
1 teaspoon clear honey
2 avocados
¼ watermelon, peeled, deseeded and chopped into bite-sized pieces
300 g (10 oz) cooked peeled king prawns
small handful of coriander leaves, chopped

1 Place the onion, garlic, chilli, lime juice and honey in a large salad bowl and mix together. Leave to stand for 10 minutes.

2 When ready to serve, halve, stone and peel the avocados, then chop the flesh and add to the salad bowl with the remaining ingredients. Toss together well and serve immediately.

PRAWN CAESAR SALAD

This classic recipe is such a great lunchtime dish, and you can use prawns, chicken, turkey, eggs or even just leaves if you are feeling very pure!

SERVES 4
PREPARATION TIME 10 MINUTES

2 cos lettuce, roughly torn
8 anchovy fillets
300 g (10 oz) cooked peeled
  king prawns

FOR THE DRESSING
juice of ½ lemon
1 large egg
1 garlic clove, crushed
2 teaspoons wholegrain mustard
2 anchovy fillets
100 ml (3½ fl oz) extra-virgin
  olive oil

1 To make the dressing, place the lemon juice, egg, garlic, mustard and anchovies in a small food processor or blender and blend together. With the motor still running, slowly add the oil through the feeder tube until the dressing starts to thicken.

2 Place the lettuce, anchovies and prawns in a serving bowl, then pour over the dressing. Lightly toss together and serve.

FIG AND HAM SALAD

With its mouthwatering combination of sweet figs and slightly salty Parma ham, this salad is simple, yet delicious.

SERVES 2
PREPARATION TIME 5 MINUTES

60 g (2¼ oz) mixed salad leaves
8 basil leaves
4 figs, halved
4 slices of Parma ham
6 cherry plum tomatoes, halved
1 tablespoon pecan nuts

FOR THE DRESSING
3 tablespoons olive oil
juice of ½ lemon
½ teaspoon wholegrain mustard
½ teaspoon clear honey

1 To make the dressing, whisk together all the ingredients in a small bowl.

2 Toss the salad leaves and basil together, then divide between 2 plates. Top each one with 2 halved figs and 2 slices of ham.

3 Scatter over the tomato halves and pecans, then drizzle with the dressing and serve.

HONEY AND MUSTARD CHICKEN SALAD

This is an easy way to create a deliciously sweet and sticky chicken dish.

SERVES 4
PREPARATION TIME 10 MINUTES
COOKING TIME 10–12 MINUTES

3 boneless, skinless chicken
    breasts, about 150 g (5 oz) each
2 tablespoons pumpkin seeds
75 g (3 oz) watercress
25 g (1 oz) rocket leaves
1 red pepper, cored, deseeded and
    thinly sliced
1 large avocado

FOR THE DRESSING
3 tablespoons olive oil
1 teaspoon clear honey
1 teaspoon Dijon mustard
1 teaspoon lemon juice

1 To make the dressing, whisk together all the ingredients in a small bowl. Set aside.

2 Cook the chicken breasts under a preheated hot grill for 5–6 minutes on each side, or until cooked through.

3 Meanwhile, heat a dry nonstick frying pan over a medium-low heat and dry-fry the pumpkin seeds for 2–3 minutes, shaking the pan occasionally, until golden and toasted.

4 Toss together the watercress and rocket and place on a serving plate. Scatter over the red pepper.

5 Halve, stone and peel the avocado, then slice the flesh. Slice the chicken diagonally and scatter over the salad leaves, then top with the avocado.

6 Sprinkle with the toasted pumpkin seeds and dressing. Serve immediately.

CRISPY DUCK AND CASHEW SALAD

Duck has a lot of fat on it, but if cooked in the right way, it can have crisp skin and tender meat with lots of flavour.

SERVES 2
PREPARATION TIME 15 MINUTES, PLUS MARINATING
COOKING TIME 7–9 MINUTES

1 teaspoon sesame oil
1 teaspoon clear honey
1 teaspoon grated fresh root ginger
1 duck breast, about 150 g (5 oz), cut into strips
1 tablespoon cashew nuts
juice of ½ lemon
1 pak choi, chopped
1 carrot, peeled and grated
2 spring onions, sliced
¼ cucumber, cut into matchsticks
25 g (1 oz) bean sprouts

1 Mix together the oil, honey and ginger in a bowl, then add the duck strips and coat well. Leave to marinate for 5 minutes.

2 Meanwhile, heat a dry nonstick frying pan over a medium-low heat and dry-fry the cashews for 3–4 minutes, shaking the pan occasionally, until golden brown and toasted. Set aside.

3 Heat a frying pan or griddle pan until hot, add the duck strips and cook for 4–5 minutes until crisp and golden.

4 Meanwhile, stir the lemon juice into the remaining marinade to make a dressing.

5 Place the remaining ingredients in a large serving bowl and toss together, then top with the duck. Serve drizzled with the dressing.

SUPERFOOD SALAD

• •

This salad has so many lovely textures and tastes and, on top of all that, it is bursting with goodness.

• •

SERVES 4
PREPARATION TIME 15 MINUTES,
  PLUS COOLING
COOKING TIME 15–18 MINUTES

500 g (1 lb) butternut squash, peeled, deseeded and chopped into 1 cm (½ inch) cubes
1 tablespoon olive oil
1 teaspoon cumin seeds
1 head of broccoli, cut into florets
200 g (7 oz) frozen or fresh peas
4 tablespoons mixed seeds, such as sunflower, pumpkin and sesame seeds
100 g (3½ oz) red cabbage, shredded
4 tomatoes, chopped
4 cooked beetroot, cut into wedges
20 g (¾ oz) alfalfa sprouts

FOR THE DRESSING
1 tablespoon olive oil
2 tablespoons avocado oil
juice of 1 lemon
½ teaspoon clear honey
½ teaspoon wholegrain mustard

1 Place the squash in a roasting tin and sprinkle with the olive oil and cumin seeds. Place in a preheated oven, 200°C (400°F), Gas Mark 6, for 15–18 minutes until tender. Remove from the roasting tin and leave to cool slightly.

2 Meanwhile, cook the broccoli and peas in a saucepan of boiling water for 4–5 minutes until tender. Drain, then refresh under cold running water and drain again.

3 Heat a dry nonstick frying pan over a medium-low heat and dry-fry the seeds for 2–3 minutes, shaking the pan occasionally, until golden brown and toasted. Leave to cool.

4 To make the dressing, place all the ingredients in a small bowl and whisk together.

5 Place the cooled squash, drained broccoli and peas and toasted seeds in a salad bowl, add the remaining ingredients, except the alfalfa sprouts, and toss together with the dressing. Serve the salad topped with the alfalfa sprouts.

ROASTED BEETROOT, WATERCRESS AND ORANGE SALAD

Beetroot is great for supporting the detoxification process so, when trying to lose weight, it's good to include it in your diet.

SERVES 4
PREPARATION TIME 15 MINUTES, PLUS COOLING
COOKING TIME 15–20 MINUTES

2 raw beetroot, peeled and chopped
½ tablespoon olive oil
½ teaspoon cumin seeds
80 g (3 oz) watercress
2 oranges, pith removed and segmented
1 large carrot, peeled and grated
25g (1 oz) pecan nuts, roughly broken

FOR THE DRESSING
2 tablespoons olive oil
1 tablespoon lemon juice
1 teaspoon clear honey
½ teaspoon wholegrain mustard
½ teaspoon chopped rosemary
freshly ground black pepper

1 Place the beetroot in a roasting tin and sprinkle with the oil and cumin seeds. Roast in a preheated oven, 200°C (400°F), Gas Mark 6, for 15–20 minutes until tender. Leave to cool slightly.

2 To make the dressing, place all the ingredients in a small bowl and whisk together.

3 Place the watercress, orange segments, grated carrot and warm roasted beetroot in a bowl, pour over the dressing and toss together, then divide among 4 plates. Sprinkle over the pecans and serve.

CRUNCHY INDIAN SALAD

These flavours are typical of Kerala in India and using ginger and lime brings out the freshness of the mango. You could serve it with freshly cooked prawns or grilled chicken.

SERVES 2
PREPARATION TIME 10 MINUTES
COOKING TIME 1–2 MINUTES

2 tablespoons sesame seeds
1 red pepper, cored, deseeded and finely sliced
3 spring onions, shredded
1 ripe mango, peeled, stoned and cut into matchsticks
25 g (1 oz) watercress

FOR THE DRESSING
2 cm (¾ inch) piece of fresh root ginger, grated
grated rind and juice of 1 lime
1 teaspoon clear honey
3 tablespoons extra-virgin olive oil
freshly ground black pepper

1 Heat a dry nonstick frying pan over a medium-low heat and dry-fry the sesame seeds for 1–2 minutes, shaking the pan occasionally, until golden brown and toasted. Set aside.

2 To make the dressing, place all the ingredients in a small bowl and whisk together.

3 Place the toasted seeds with the remaining ingredients in a large bowl and toss together, then pour over the dressing and toss again before serving.

CHUNKY CUMIN WALDORF SALAD

Waldorf salad has been around since the 1890s and was first created in New York. This Paleo version just adds a little bit of spice and omits the mayonnaise.

SERVES 4
PREPARATION TIME 10 MINUTES
COOKING TIME 3–4 MINUTES

60 g (2¼ oz) walnut pieces
100 g (3½ oz) green grapes, halved
6 celery sticks, sliced diagonally
1 green dessert apple, peeled,
   cored and thinly sliced

FOR THE DRESSING
50 g (2 oz) ground almonds
100 ml (3½ fl oz) non-dairy milk
1 teaspoon ground cumin

1 Heat a dry nonstick frying pan over a medium-low heat and dry-fry the walnuts for 3–4 minutes, shaking the pan occasionally, until golden brown and toasted. Set aside.

2 To make the dressing, place all the ingredients in a small food processor or blender and blend together.

3 Transfer the dressing to a large bowl, then add the toasted walnuts, grapes, celery and apple and toss well to coat.

4 Serve immediately, or cover and chill until required.

PALEO TABBOULEH

Who would have thought parsnips could be a good substitute for bulgur wheat? This has a much crunchier texture than traditional tabbouleh, but is very tasty.

SERVES 4
PREPARATION TIME 10 MINUTES,
PLUS STANDING
COOKING TIME 2–3 MINUTES

30 g (1¼ oz) pine nuts
1 parsnip, peeled and roughly
    chopped
small handful of parsley
small handful of basil leaves
small handful of coriander leaves
¼ cucumber, diced
juice of ½ lemon
1 tablespoon extra-virgin olive oil
freshly ground black pepper

1 Heat a dry nonstick frying pan over a medium-low heat and dry-fry the pine nuts for 2–3 minutes, shaking the pan occasionally, until golden brown and toasted. Set aside.

2 Place the parsnip in a food processor and blitz until broken down into coarse crumbs. Add the toasted pine nuts and herbs and process until the mixture resembles bulgur wheat.

3 Transfer the mixture to a bowl, stir in the remaining ingredients and season with pepper. Leave to stand for at least 5 minutes to allow the flavours to develop.

CRUNCHY KALE SALAD

This flavour-packed salad is great to take to work or on a picnic as it doesn't wilt.

SERVES 2
PREPARATION TIME 10 MINUTES
COOKING TIME 3–4 MINUTES

50 g (2 oz) walnut halves
50 g (2 oz) kale, thinly shredded
1 carrot, peeled and cut into thin strips
1 small raw beetroot, peeled and cut into thin strips

FOR THE DRESSING
grated rind and juice of 1 lemon
1 tablespoon extra-virgin olive oil
½ teaspoon sesame oil
freshly ground black pepper

1 Heat a dry nonstick frying pan over a medium-low heat and dry-fry the walnuts for 3–4 minutes, shaking the pan occasionally, until golden brown and toasted. Set aside.

2 To make the dressing, whisk together all the ingredients in a small bowl. Place the kale, carrot and beetroot in a bowl, pour over the dressing and toss together.

3 Serve the salad sprinkled with the toasted walnuts.

ORANGE, AVOCADO AND CASHEW SALAD

This refreshing salad is really quick and easy to make – just the thing when you want to whip up a meal for one.

SERVES 1
PREPARATION TIME 10 MINUTES
COOKING TIME 3–4 MINUTES

2 tablespoons cashew nuts
1 orange
1 avocado
25 g (1 oz) watercress
1 tablespoon olive oil

1 Heat a dry nonstick frying pan over a medium-low heat and dry-fry the cashews for 3–4 minutes, shaking the pan occasionally, until golden brown and toasted. Set aside.

2 Meanwhile, using a sharp knife, remove the peel and pith from the orange. Hold the orange over a bowl to catch the juice and cut out the segments. Place the orange segments in a separate bowl.

3 Halve, stone and peel the avocado, then chop the flesh. Add to the orange segments and mix together. Toss the watercress into the bowl.

4 Transfer the salad to a serving plate and sprinkle with the toasted cashews.

5 Add the oil to the reserved orange juice and whisk together. Drizzle over the salad and serve.

GINGER, MANGETOUT AND BEAN SPROUT COLESLAW

Not all coleslaw has to be cabbage! This tasty version uses other crunchy veg, with some spice to liven it up.

SERVES 4
PREPARATION TIME 15 MINUTES, PLUS COOLING
COOKING TIME 3–4 MINUTES

50 g (2 oz) hazelnuts
75 g (3 oz) mangetout, thinly shredded
90 g (3¾ oz) bean sprouts
1 red pepper, cored, deseeded and thinly sliced
5 radishes, thinly sliced

FOR THE DRESSING
2 tablespoons olive oil
1 tablespoon lemon juice
1 teaspoon toasted sesame oil
½ lemon grass stalk, outer leaves discarded and finely diced
2 cm (¾ inch) piece of fresh root ginger, peeled and finely diced
1 teaspoon coconut palm sugar

1 Heat a dry nonstick frying pan over a medium-low heat and dry-fry the hazelnuts for 3–4 minutes, shaking the pan occasionally, until golden brown and toasted. Leave to cool slightly, then roughly chop and set aside.

2 To make the dressing, place all the ingredients in a small bowl and whisk together until the sugar has dissolved and the dressing has emulsified.

3 Place the toasted nuts and the remaining ingredients in a large bowl, then pour over the dressing and toss together to serve.

4

FISH AND SEAFOOD

HONEY AND WASABI-GLAZED SALMON FILLETS

Wasabi is a hot paste that adds great flavour and heat to this dish so use sparingly!

SERVES 2
PREPARATION TIME 5 MINUTES
COOKING TIME 8 MINUTES

juice of 1 lemon
1 tablespoon clear honey
1 teaspoon grated fresh root
   ginger
½–1 teaspoon wasabi paste
1 tablespoon sesame seeds
2 teaspoons coconut oil
2 salmon fillets, about 150 g
   (5 oz) each
crisp green salad, to serve

1 Place the lemon juice, honey, ginger and wasabi paste in a small saucepan and gently heat together. Bring to a simmer, then remove from the heat.

2 Meanwhile, heat a dry nonstick frying pan over a medium-low heat and dry-fry the sesame seeds for 1–2 minutes, shaking the pan occasionally, until golden and toasted. Set aside.

3 Heat the oil in a separate frying pan or griddle pan, add the salmon, skin side up, and cook for 3 minutes. Turn the fish over and cook for a further 2 minutes, or until the fish is cooked through.

4 Pour over the glaze, sprinkle with the toasted sesame seeds and cook for a further minute. Serve with a crisp green salad.

GRILLED SALMON WITH AVOCADO SALSA

Both salmon and avocado are rich in essential fats, so it's very important to include them in your diet.

SERVES 2
PREPARATION TIME 10 MINUTES
COOKING TIME 6–8 MINUTES

2 salmon steaks, about 150 g (5 oz) each
25 g (1 oz) watercress or rocket leaves

FOR THE SALSA
1 avocado
2 spring onions, sliced
10 cherry tomatoes, quartered
1 tablespoon chopped coriander
juice of ½ lime
½ teaspoon sesame oil

1 To make the salsa, halve, stone and peel the avocado, then dice the flesh. Place in a non-metallic bowl, add the remaining ingredients and mix together. Leave to stand while you cook the salmon.

2 Cook the salmon under a preheated hot grill for 3–4 minutes on each side, or until the fish is cooked through.

3 Divide the watercress or rocket between 2 plates and top with the salmon. Spoon over the salsa and serve.

SALMON AND GRAPEFRUIT CEVICHE

If you love sushi or sashimi, you will enjoy ceviche – the fish is 'cooked' by the acidity of the grapefruit juice, which makes it beautifully tender, too.

SERVES 4
PREPARATION TIME 10 MINUTES, PLUS MARINATING

1 grapefruit
juice of 1 lime
1 red chilli, deseeded and thinly sliced
4 spring onions, sliced
1 tablespoon chopped coriander
500 g (1 lb) skinless salmon fillet, thinly sliced
crisp salad leaves, to serve

1 Cut the grapefruit in half. Squeeze the juice from one of the halves and pour into a non-metallic bowl. Using a sharp knife, cut the pith from the remaining half and cut out the segments, then chop and add to the bowl. Stir in the lime juice, chilli, spring onions and coriander.

2 Place the salmon in the marinade and mix well. Cover and leave to marinate in the refrigerator for 30 minutes.

3 Arrange the salmon slices on a bed of crisp salad leaves and serve.

GRILLED SALMON WITH COCONUT CABBAGE

If you prefer a spicy version, simply add finely diced red chilli to this Indian-inspired recipe.

SERVES 4
PREPARATION TIME 5 MINUTES
COOKING TIME 10–12 MINUTES

1 tablespoon coconut oil
2 teaspoons cumin seeds
1 onion, sliced
½ teaspoon turmeric
½ large Savoy cabbage, shredded
1 tablespoon desiccated coconut
2 tablespoons water
4 salmon fillets, about 150 g (5 oz) each
freshly ground black pepper

1 Heat the oil in a large frying pan, add the cumin seeds and onion and cook for 3–4 minutes until the onion is starting to soften. Stir in the turmeric and cook for a further minute.

2 Add the cabbage and coconut and toss to coat with the spices. Add the measurement water and bring to a simmer, then cover and cook for 5–6 minutes.

3 Meanwhile, cook the salmon under a preheated hot grill for 3–4 minutes on each side, or until the fish is cooked through.

4 Uncover the cabbage, toss and season with pepper, then serve with the grilled salmon.

THAI SEA BASS EN PAPILLOTE

Cooking fish wrapped in greaseproof paper helps to seal in the flavours and ensure the fish stays moist, too. Ask your fishmonger to scale and gut the fish.

SERVES 2
PREPARATION TIME 15 MINUTES
COOKING TIME 20–25 MINUTES

75 g (3 oz) fresh root ginger, peeled and sliced
2 lemon grass stalks, outer leaves discarded and sliced
2 garlic cloves, peeled and bruised
1 red chilli, deseeded and finely diced
grated rind and juice of 1 lime
2 small sea bass, about 500 g (1 lb) each, scaled and gutted
freshly ground black pepper
small handful of coriander leaves, to garnish

1 Mix together the ginger, lemon grass, garlic, chilli and lime rind and juice in a bowl, then fill the cavities of the fish with three-quarters of the mixture.

2 Place each fish on a large piece of greaseproof paper, sprinkle over the remaining stuffing mixture and season with pepper. Fold up the sides of the paper to seal the parcels and place on a baking sheet.

3 Bake in a preheated oven, 180°C (350°F), Gas Mark 4, for 20–25 minutes until the fish is cooked through and the flesh flakes off the bone.

4 Serve the fish sprinkled with coriander leaves.

GRILLED RED MULLET AND ROASTED FENNEL WITH CHILLI OIL

Fennel is the perfect accompaniment to fish and, if you can't find red mullet, this recipe works well with sea bream, too.

SERVES 2
PREPARATION TIME 10 MINUTES, PLUS STANDING
COOKING TIME 35 MINUTES

2 fennel bulbs, trimmed and sliced
1 tablespoon olive oil
4 red mullet fillets, about 150–175 g (5–6 oz) each

FOR THE CHILLI OIL
2 garlic cloves, finely chopped
1 teaspoon chilli flakes
75 ml (3 fl oz) olive oil
2 tablespoons chopped parsley

1 To make the chilli oil, place the garlic, chilli flakes and oil in a small saucepan and heat very gently for 5 minutes. Remove from the heat and leave to stand while you cook the fennel.

2 Place the fennel in a roasting tin and drizzle with the oil. Place in a preheated oven, 200°C (400°F), Gas Mark 6, for 30 minutes until the fennel is tender.

3 Towards the end of the cooking time, cook the fish under a preheated hot grill for 3–4 minutes on each side, or until the fish is cooked through.

4 Stir the parsley into the chilli oil. Spoon the fennel on to 2 warmed plates, top with the fish and serve drizzled with the chilli oil.

PANCETTA-WRAPPED MONKFISH

Monkfish is a solid, meaty fish. Ask your fishmonger to remove the outer membrane of the tail as this can be difficult to do.

SERVES 4
PREPARATION TIME 5 MINUTES,
**   PLUS RESTING**
COOKING TIME 16–20 MINUTES

400 g (13 oz) monkfish tail, sliced
    in half lengthways
150 g (5 oz) pancetta slices
1 tablespoon thyme leaves
steamed purple sprouting broccoli,
    to serve

1 Lay the monkfish halves together in opposite directions, so that a thick and a thin end are together at both ends.

2 Lay the pancetta slices on a board, slightly overlapping, then place the monkfish in the centre and sprinkle over the thyme. Wrap the pancetta around the fish to enclose it completely.

3 Cook under a preheated hot grill for 8–10 minutes on each side, or until the fish is cooked through. Leave to rest for 2–3 minutes.

4 Slice the fish into medallions and serve with steamed purple sprouting broccoli.

PAN-FRIED COD WITH MINTED PEA PURÉE

Peas and mint are a great combination. You can serve the pea purée with other fish or seafood. It works particularly well with scallops.

SERVES 2
PREPARATION TIME 10 MINUTES
COOKING TIME 8–11 MINUTES

1 tablespoon olive oil
2 cod fillets, about 150 g (5 oz) each
1 tablespoon chopped chives, to garnish

FOR THE PURÉE
250 g (8 oz) frozen peas
6–8 mint leaves, chopped
1 tablespoon non-dairy milk
freshly ground black pepper

1 To make the purée, cook the peas in a saucepan of boiling water for 2–3 minutes, then drain and place in a food processor or blender with the mint, milk and some pepper. Blend until smooth. Alternatively, for a more rustic purée, drain the peas and return to the pan, then mash. Set aside and keep warm.

2 Heat the oil in a frying pan, add the cod and cook for 3–4 minutes on each side, until the fish is cooked through.

3 Divide the pea purée between 2 warmed plates, top with the cod and serve sprinkled with the chopped chives.

ORANGE AND TOMATO ROASTED COD

Adding orange to this dish gives it a real lift. You can ring the changes by using lemon, too.

SERVES 4
PREPARATION TIME 10 MINUTES
COOKING TIME 45–50 MINUTES

500 g (1 lb) plum tomatoes, quartered
2 onions, cut into wedges
rind of 1 orange, cut into julienne strips
1 tablespoon thyme leaves
1 tablespoon olive oil
4 cod loins, about 150 g (5 oz) each
2 tablespoons flaked almonds
freshly ground black pepper
crisp green salad or steamed green vegetables, to serve

1 Place the tomatoes, onions, orange strips, thyme and oil in a roasting tin, season with pepper and mix well. Roast in a preheated oven, 200°C (400°F), Gas Mark 6, for 35–40 minutes, stirring once, until the onions start to caramelize.

2 Increase the oven temperature to 220°C (425°F), Gas Mark 7. Remove the tin from the oven, nestle the cod loins in the vegetables, spooning some over the fish. Sprinkle over the flaked almonds.

3 Return to the oven and roast for 10–12 minutes until the cod is cooked through. Serve with a crisp green salad or steamed greens.

GRILLED COD WITH PESTO BEANS

Shop-bought pesto includes Parmesan, which is not allowed on the Paleo diet. The pesto in this recipe is just as delicious, and you could make a bigger batch of it and store in the refrigerator for a few days.

SERVES 2
PREPARATION TIME 10 MINUTES, PLUS COOLING
COOKING TIME 8–11 MINUTES

2 cod loins, about 150 g (5 oz) each
150 g (5 oz) green beans, trimmed

FOR THE PESTO
2 tablespoons pine nuts
large handful of basil leaves
1 small garlic clove, chopped
3–4 tablespoons olive oil

1 To make the pesto, heat a dry nonstick frying pan over a medium-low heat and dry-fry the pine nuts for 2–3 minutes, shaking the pan occasionally, until golden brown and toasted. Leave to cool.

2 Place the basil, toasted pine nuts and garlic in a small food processor or blender and blitz until broken down. With the motor still running, slowly add the oil through the feeder tube until it forms a loose paste. Set aside.

3 Cook the cod under a preheated hot grill for 3–4 minutes on each side, or until the fish is cooked through.

4 Meanwhile, put the green beans in a steamer, cover and cook for 3–4 minutes until just tender.

5 Toss the green beans in the pesto, then divide between 2 warmed plates. Top with the grilled cod and serve.

GRILLED COD WITH PEPERONATA

Peperonata is a traditional Italian dish of sweet peppers and onions that can be served on its own or to accompany grilled fish.

SERVES 4
PREPARATION TIME 15 MINUTES
COOKING TIME 45 MINUTES

500 g (1 lb) ripe tomatoes
4 tablespoons olive oil
2 onions, chopped
2 garlic cloves, crushed
4 red peppers, cored, deseeded
    and thickly sliced
2 yellow peppers, cored, deseeded
    and thickly sliced
6–8 basil leaves, roughly torn
4 cod loins, about 150 g (5 oz)
    each
freshly ground black pepper

1 Place the tomatoes in a heatproof bowl and pour over boiling water to cover. Leave for 1–2 minutes, then drain, cut a cross at the stem end of each tomato and peel off the skins. Chop the flesh and set aside.

2 Heat the oil in a large frying pan, add the onions and garlic and cook for 4–5 minutes, stirring occasionally, until softened. Add the peppers and cook over a medium heat for a further 12 minutes.

3 Stir in the tomatoes and basil, season with pepper and continue to cook for 30 minutes, stirring occasionally.

4 Towards the end of the cooking time, cook the cod under a preheated hot grill for 3–4 minutes on each side, or until the fish is cooked through. Serve the cod on the peperonata.

MUSHROOM-STUFFED TROUT

This looks very impressive, but is actually simple to make and tastes delicious.

SERVES 4
PREPARATION TIME 15 MINUTES
COOKING TIME 35–40 MINUTES

2 tablespoons olive oil
1 onion, finely chopped
1 garlic clove, crushed
300 g (10 oz) chestnut mushrooms, chopped
150 g (5 oz) flaked almonds
2 tablespoons chopped coriander
2 whole trout, about 700–800 g (1½–1¾ lb) each, cleaned and gutted
freshly ground black pepper
steamed broccoli, to serve

1 Heat the oil in a frying pan, add the onion and cook for 4–5 minutes until softened. Add the garlic and mushrooms and cook for a further 6–8 minutes until the mushrooms are tender. Remove from the heat, add the flaked almonds and coriander and mix well.

2 Season the fish with pepper inside and out, then stuff with the mushroom filling. Wrap each one loosely in foil and place on a baking sheet.

3 Bake in a preheated oven, 200°C (400°F), Gas Mark 6, for 25 minutes, or until the fish is just cooked through. Serve with steamed broccoli.

MACKEREL CURRY

Mackerel is one of the oily fish that are rich in omega-3 essential fats – vital for a healthy diet.

SERVES 4
PREPARATION TIME 10 MINUTES
COOKING TIME 16–20 MINUTES

1 tablespoon coconut oil
1 teaspoon cumin seeds
1 large onion, sliced
150 ml (¼ pint) coconut milk
250 ml (8 fl oz) water
450 g (14½ oz) fresh mackerel
    fillets, skinned and cut into 5 cm
    (2 inch) pieces
small handful of coriander leaves,
    roughly torn
freshly ground black pepper

FOR THE CURRY PASTE
1 green chilli, deseeded and chopped
1 teaspoon ground coriander
½ teaspoon turmeric
4 garlic cloves
2.5 cm (1 inch) piece of fresh root ginger,
    peeled and chopped
1 teaspoon coconut oil

TO SERVE
wilted spinach leaves
lemon wedges

1 To make the curry paste, place all the ingredients in a small food processor or blender and blend until smooth.

2 Heat the oil in a wok or frying pan, add the paste and the cumin seeds and cook for 2–3 minutes. Add the onion and cook for a further 1–2 minutes until starting to soften.

3 Pour in the coconut milk and measurement water and bring to the boil, then reduce the heat and simmer for 5 minutes. Season with pepper.

4 Add the mackerel to the pan and cook for 6–8 minutes until the fish is cooked through. Stir in the coriander leaves.

5 Serve the curry with wilted spinach and lemon wedges.

GINGER AND ORANGE MACKEREL WITH COLESLAW

Here, coleslaw gets its creaminess from a delicious cashew nut dressing.

SERVES 4
PREPARATION TIME 20 MINUTES, PLUS MARINATING
COOKING TIME 25–30 MINUTES

4 fresh mackerel fillets, about
    150 g (5 oz) each
juice of 2 oranges
grated rind of 1 orange
1 teaspoon grated fresh root
    ginger
2 teaspoons tomato purée

FOR THE COLESLAW
50 g (2 oz) cashew nuts
2 spring onions, chopped
juice of ½ lemon
½ teaspoon clear honey
¼ red cabbage, shredded
¼ white cabbage, shredded
2 carrots, peeled and grated
small handful of coriander leaves

1 Place the mackerel fillets in a non-metallic ovenproof dish. Mix together the orange juice, orange rind, ginger and tomato purée in a small bowl, then pour over the mackerel. Cover and leave to marinate in the refrigerator for at least 30 minutes.

2 To make the dressing for the coleslaw, place the cashews, spring onions, lemon juice and honey in a food processor or blender and blend until smooth, gradually adding enough water to form the consistency of thick double cream.

3 Mix together the cabbages, carrots and coriander in a large bowl, then pour over the dressing and toss together. Leave to stand while you cook the mackerel.

4 Cover the mackerel in the dish with foil and bake in a preheated oven, 200°C (400°F), Gas Mark 6, for 25–30 minutes until the fish is cooked through. Serve with the coleslaw.

MACKEREL FILLETS WITH FENNEL COLESLAW

Mackerel is quick to cook in a frying pan or griddle pan and also great cooked over a barbecue.

SERVES 4
PREPARATION TIME 15 MINUTES
COOKING TIME 4–6 MINUTES

1 tablespoon olive oil
4 fresh mackerel fillets, about
    150 g (5 oz) each

FOR THE COLESLAW
2 tablespoons olive oil
juice of ½ lemon
1 teaspoon clear honey
½ teaspoon wholegrain mustard
10 g (⅓ oz) dill, chopped
2 celery sticks, thinly sliced
½ cucumber, thinly sliced
1 fennel bulb, trimmed and thinly
    sliced
freshly ground black pepper
    (optional)

1 To make the dressing for the coleslaw, whisk together the oil, lemon juice, honey, mustard and dill in a small bowl. Season with pepper, if liked.

2 Mix together the celery, cucumber and fennel in a large bowl, then pour over the dressing and toss together. Leave to stand while you cook the mackerel.

3 Heat the oil in a frying pan or griddle pan, add the mackerel and cook for 2–3 minutes on each side, or until the fish is cooked through. Alternatively, cook the fish on a barbecue.

4 Divide the coleslaw among 4 plates, top with the mackerel and serve.

LEMON AND PARSLEY SARDINES

Containing omega-3 essential fats and calcium, sardines are cheap and good for you. And if it's a sunny day, you can cook them on the barbecue.

SERVES 4
PREPARATION TIME 10 MINUTES
COOKING TIME 6–8 MINUTES

4–8 sardines, depending on their size
2 lemons
1 tablespoon olive oil
25g (1 oz) flaked almonds
freshly ground black pepper
1 tablespoon chopped parsley, to garnish

1 Wash the sardines to remove all the scales, then slash each side a couple of times using a sharp knife.

2 Squeeze the juice from 1 of the lemons, then rub this all over the sardines, especially into the cuts, with the pepper.

3 Heat the oil in a frying pan or griddle pan. Cut the remaining lemon into wedges and add to the pan. Add the sardines and cook for 3–4 minutes on each side, or until the fish is cooked through.

4 Meanwhile, heat a dry nonstick frying pan over a medium-low heat and dry-fry the flaked almonds for 2–3 minutes, shaking the pan occasionally, until golden brown and toasted.

5 Serve the sardines sprinkled with the toasted almonds and the parsley.

TUNA CARPACCIO

Ask your fishmonger for the freshest fish he has, from a sustainable source, for this raw fish recipe.

SERVES 4
PREPARATION TIME 15 MINUTES

400 g (13 oz) fresh tuna
4 radishes, thinly sliced
¼ cucumber, thinly sliced
4 spring onions, thinly sliced
juice of 1 lime
1 tablespoon extra-virgin olive oil
freshly ground black pepper

1 Using a very sharp knife, cut the tuna into very thin strips, then place on a large serving plate.

2 Scatter the radishes, cucumber and spring onions around the plate, then sprinkle with the lime juice, olive oil and pepper. Serve immediately.

FISH TAGINE

This is a fragrant fish dish based on the spices used in Morocco. Try it with haddock, cod or any white fish of your choice.

SERVES 4
PREPARATION TIME 15 MINUTES, PLUS MARINATING
COOKING TIME 25–30 MINUTES

4 haddock or cod fillets, about
    150 g (5 oz) each
1 tablespoon olive oil
1 large onion, sliced
2 garlic cloves, roughly chopped
1 teaspoon ground cumin
1 teaspoon paprika
400 g (13 oz) can chopped
    tomatoes
300 ml (½ pint) fish stock
grated rind of 1 lemon
2 red peppers, cored, deseeded
    and chopped
½ small bunch of coriander,
    chopped
juice of ½ lemon

FOR THE MARINADE
1 tablespoon olive oil
2 garlic cloves, roughly chopped
1 teaspoon ground cumin
1 teaspoon paprika
½ small bunch of coriander
juice of ½ lemon

1 To make the marinade, place all the ingredients in a small food processor or blender and blend until smooth. Place the fish in a non-metallic dish, and spoon over the marinade. Cover and leave to marinate in the refrigerator.

2 Meanwhile, heat the oil in a large saucepan, add the onion and garlic and cook for 4–5 minutes until softened. Stir in the cumin and paprika and cook for a further 2 minutes.

3 Stir in the tomatoes, stock and lemon rind and simmer for 8–10 minutes. Add the peppers, cover and continue to cook for 5–6 minutes until the peppers start to soften.

4 Stir in the chopped coriander, then place the fish on top, cover and cook for 4–6 minutes, or until the fish is cooked through. Serve drizzled with the lemon juice.

FISH STEW

You can use any meaty fish for this stew –
pollock, cod, tilapia, or even salmon all work well.

SERVES 4
PREPARATION TIME 10 MINUTES
COOKING TIME 16–20 MINUTES

1 tablespoon olive oil
1 onion, chopped
2 garlic cloves, crushed
1 teaspoon ground cumin
½ teaspoon paprika
400 g (13 oz) can chopped
    tomatoes
200 ml (7 fl oz) fish stock
1 red pepper, cored, deseeded
    and chopped
500 g (1 lb) skinless fish fillets,
    cut into large chunks
125 g (4 oz) cooked peeled king
    prawns
small handful of coriander leaves
lemon wedges, to serve

1 Heat the oil in a large saucepan, add the onion, garlic, cumin and paprika and cook for 3-4 minutes until the onion is softened.

2 Add the tomatoes, stock and red pepper and bring to a simmer, then cook for 8–10 minutes.

3 Add the fish and prawns to the tomato mixture and cook for a further 4–5 minutes until the fish is cooked through.

4 Stir in the coriander and serve with lemon wedges.

SQUID WITH TOMATOES

Squid is now easy to find, but ask your fishmonger to prepare it for you as it has a tough outer skin that needs to be removed.

SERVES 4
PREPARATION TIME 10 MINUTES
COOKING TIME 20–25 MINUTES

1 tablespoon olive oil
1 red onion, diced
2 garlic cloves, chopped
1 red chilli, deseeded and finely diced
pinch of paprika
400 g (13 oz) can chopped tomatoes
500 g (1 lb) fresh squid, cut into rings
grated rind of 1 lemon
small handful of parsley leaves
freshly ground black pepper

1 Heat the oil in a frying pan, add the onion, garlic and chilli and cook for 2–3 minutes until starting to soften.

2 Stir in the paprika, then pour in the tomatoes. Bring to the boil, then reduce the heat and simmer for 12–15 minutes.

3 Add the squid to the pan, cover and cook for 5 minutes until the squid is tender and cooked through.

4 Stir in the lemon rind and parsley, season with pepper and serve.

TOMATO AND CHILLI MUSSELS

Mussels are cheap, sustainable and delightfully simple to cook.

SERVES 2
PREPARATION TIME 20 MINUTES
COOKING TIME 7–10 MINUTES

2 tomatoes
2 tablespoons olive oil
2 garlic cloves, chopped
1 shallot, diced
1 red chilli, deseeded and finely diced
200 ml (7 fl oz) water
1 teaspoon tomato purée
1 kg (2 lb) mussels, scrubbed and debearded (discard any with broken shells or that don't close when tapped)
freshly ground black pepper
handful of basil leaves, roughly torn, to garnish

1 Place the tomatoes in a heatproof bowl and pour over boiling water to cover. Leave for 1–2 minutes, then drain, cut a cross at the stem end of each tomato and peel off the skins. Halve and deseed, then roughly chop the flesh.

2 Heat the oil in a large saucepan that has a tight-fitting lid, add the garlic, shallot and chilli and cook for 2–3 minutes until starting to soften. Stir in the measurement water and tomato purée, then season with pepper. Simmer for 1–2 minutes.

3 Add the mussels and give them a stir. Cover the pan tightly and leave to cook for 3–4 minutes, shaking the pan a couple of times, until all the shells have opened. Discard any mussels that remain shut.

4 Divide between 2 warmed bowls and serve sprinkled with the basil.

CRAB AND SWEET POTATO CAKES

These are delicious and can be made in advance and chilled until you want to cook them. They are perfect as a packed lunch or to take on a picnic.

SERVES 4
PREPARATION TIME 20 MINUTES, PLUS COOLING
COOKING TIME 20–30 MINUTES

350 g (11½ oz) sweet potatoes, peeled and chopped
1 tablespoon olive oil
350 g (11½ oz) crabmeat, a mixture of dark and white
¼ red pepper, cored, deseeded and finely diced
2 tablespoons chopped chives
2 tablespoons coconut or almond flour
1 tablespoon coconut oil
freshly ground black pepper

1 Place the sweet potatoes in a roasting tin and toss with the olive oil, then roast in a preheated oven, 200°C (400°F), Gas Mark 6, for 15–20 minutes until tender. Transfer to a bowl and roughly mash, then leave to cool for 5–6 minutes.

2 Add the crabmeat, red pepper and chives, season with pepper and mix together until well combined. Using wet hands, shape the mixture into 8 small cakes.

3 Put the coconut or almond flour in a small bowl, then toss the potato cakes in the flour to coat.

4 Heat the coconut oil in a large frying pan, add the cakes and cook for 3–4 minutes on each side until golden. Serve hot or cold.

SPICY SEARED SCALLOPS WITH MANGO AND AVOCADO SALSA

If you like scallops, you will love this recipe where they are served with a fruity salsa on the side.

SERVES 2
PREPARATION TIME 10 MINUTES
COOKING TIME 4–6 MINUTES

6 scallops
½ tablespoon mild curry powder
1 tablespoon olive oil

FOR THE SALSA
1 small avocado
1 small mango, peeled, stoned
  and diced
¼ cucumber, diced
juice of ½ lime
1 tablespoon olive oil

1 To make the salsa, halve, stone and peel the avocado, then dice the flesh and place in a non-metallic bowl. Stir in the mango and cucumber, then drizzle over the lime juice and oil. Leave to stand while you cook the scallops.

2 Sprinkle the scallops with the curry powder. Heat the oil in a frying pan, add the scallops and cook over a high heat for 2–3 minutes on each side until just golden.

3 Divide the scallops between 2 plates and serve with spoonfuls of the salsa.

SEAFOOD STIR-FRY

If your fishmonger sells mixed seafood, you can just replace the prawns, squid and mussels with 450 g (14½ oz) of mixed seafood.

SERVES 4
PREPARATION TIME 10 MINUTES, PLUS MARINATING
COOKING TIME 7–10 MINUTES

2 teaspoons clear honey
grated rind and juice of 1 lime
24 raw peeled tiger prawns, about 250 g (8oz)
75 g (3 oz) ready-cooked squid rings
125 g (4 oz) ready-cooked shelled mussels
1 tablespoon coconut oil
1 teaspoon sesame oil
4 spring onions, sliced
1 red pepper, cored, deseeded and sliced
1 yellow pepper, cored, deseeded and sliced
150 g (5 oz) bean sprouts
150 g (5 oz) pak choi, chopped

1 Mix together the honey, lime rind and juice in a small bowl. Place the prawns, squid and mussels in a non-metallic bowl and pour over the marinade. Leave to marinate for 5 minutes.

2 Heat the oils in a wok, add the drained seafood and stir-fry for 2–3 minutes until the prawns turn pink. Remove from the pan and set aside.

3 Add the spring onions and peppers to the pan and stir-fry for 2 minutes, then add the bean sprouts and pak choi and stir-fry for a further 1–2 minutes.

4 Return the seafood to the pan and stir-fry for 2–3 minutes until piping hot. Serve immediately.

THAI GREEN PRAWN CURRY

Preparing your own Thai curry paste is easy. It tastes so much better than shop-bought and you can make it as hot as you like. The paste can be kept in the refrigerator for up to a week.

SERVES 4
**PREPARATION TIME 15 MINUTES,
    PLUS COOLING**
COOKING TIME 25–30 MINUTES

1 tablespoon coconut oil
1 aubergine, chopped
400 ml (14 fl oz) can coconut milk
100 g (3½ oz) mangetout
100 ml (3½ fl oz) fish stock
500 g (1 lb) raw peeled king prawns
grated rind and juice of 1 lime
2 tablespoons chopped coriander

FOR THE CURRY PASTE
1 teaspoon coriander seeds
1 teaspoon cumin seeds
4 green bird's-eye chillies, chopped
2.5 cm (1 inch) piece of fresh root ginger,
    peeled and chopped
4 garlic cloves, chopped
1 shallot, finely chopped
1 lemon grass stalk, outer leaves discarded
    and finely chopped
1 small bunch of coriander, including
    the stalks
2 kaffir lime leaves
1 tablespoon fish sauce

1 Heat a dry nonstick frying pan over a medium-low heat and dry-fry the coriander seeds and cumin seeds for 3–4 minutes until lightly toasted and fragrant. Leave to cool.

2 To make the curry paste, place the toasted seeds and the remaining ingredients in a food processor or blender and blend until nearly smooth. Transfer to an airtight container and store for up to 1 week in the refrigerator.

3 Heat the oil in a large frying pan or wok, add the aubergine and cook for 10–12 minutes until golden brown and softened. Stir in 2 tablespoons of the curry paste and cook for a further 3–4 minutes.

4 Pour in the coconut milk and bring to the boil, then reduce the heat to a simmer, add the mangetout and cook for a few minutes. Then add the stock and prawns and cook for 4–5 minutes until the prawns turn pink and are cooked through.

5 Stir in the lime rind and juice and chopped coriander, then ladle into 4 warmed bowls and serve.

PRAWN AND EGG STIR-FRY

Everyone loves a stir-fry – quick to make and only one pan to wash up!

SERVES 2
PREPARATION TIME 5 MINUTES
COOKING TIME 10 MINUTES

1 tablespoon coconut oil
100 g (3½ oz) cooked peeled
  prawns
2 cm (¾ inch) piece of fresh root
  ginger, grated
1 garlic clove, crushed
50 g (2 oz) bean sprouts
4 spring onions, sliced
1 pak choi, chopped
4 eggs, beaten
small handful of coriander leaves,
  roughly torn

1 Heat the oil in a wok or large frying pan, add the prawns and stir-fry for 30 seconds, then add the ginger, garlic, bean sprouts, half the spring onions and the pak choi and stir-fry for a further minute.

2 Reduce the temperature and add the eggs, leaving them to set a little before moving them around with a spatula or chopsticks until scrambled.

3 Stir in the remaining spring onions and the coriander and serve.

5

MEAT, POULTRY AND GAME

MOROCCAN BEEF KEBABS

Choose good-quality meat for this dish and, for a wonderful flavour, cook the kebabs over a barbecue.

SERVES 4
PREPARATION TIME 15 MINUTES, PLUS MARINATING
COOKING TIME 6–8 MINUTES

2 tablespoons olive oil
juice of 1 lemon
2 garlic cloves, crushed
2 tablespoons chopped coriander
2 teaspoons ground coriander
2 teaspoons ground cumin
½ teaspoon chilli flakes
¼ teaspoon ground cinnamon
750 g (1½ lb) lean steak, cut into bite-sized pieces
crisp green salad, to serve

1 Mix together the oil, lemon juice, garlic, chopped coriander and spices in a non-metallic bowl. Add the pieces of beef and toss well to coat in the spicy oil. Cover and leave to marinate in the refrigerator for 1 hour.

2 Thread the beef on to 8 metal skewers, then cook under a preheated hot grill or on a barbecue for 3–4 minutes on each side, or until browned and cooked to your liking.

3 Serve with a crisp green salad.

SPICY BEEF STIR-FRY

Use lean steak for this spicy stir-fry and vary the vegetables depending on what's in season. If you want a bit of heat, add a diced red chilli to the pan with the garlic.

SERVES 2
PREPARATION TIME 10 MINUTES
COOKING TIME 8–9 MINUTES

1 tablespoon coconut oil
250 g (8 oz) lean beef steak, cut into thin strips
2 teaspoons Chinese five-spice powder
1 garlic clove, crushed
2 cm (1 inch) piece of fresh root ginger, peeled and finely diced
4 spring onions, sliced
200 g (7 oz) spring greens, shredded
2 tablespoons water

1 Heat the oil in a wok or large frying pan, add the beef and stir-fry for 2–3 minutes until starting to brown.

2 Add the five-spice powder, garlic and ginger and stir-fry for a further minute, then stir in the spring onions and greens.

3 Add the measurement water and stir-fry until the greens have wilted. Serve immediately.

FILLET STEAK WITH SWEET POTATO FRIES

This simple dinner recipe for two can be served with a fresh green salad if you want to add some colour to your plate.

SERVES 2
PREPARATION TIME 5 MINUTES, PLUS RESTING
COOKING TIME 18–20 MINUTES

2 sweet potatoes, scrubbed and cut into thin strips
1 tablespoon olive oil
2 lean fillet steaks, about 150 g (5 oz) each
freshly ground black pepper

1 Place the sweet potatoes on a large baking sheet. Drizzle with the oil, then sprinkle with pepper and toss well.

2 Spread the strips out in an even layer and place in a preheated oven, 200°C (400°F), Gas Mark 6, for 18–20 minutes until tender and golden.

3 Meanwhile, heat a griddle pan until hot, add the steak and cook to your liking. Leave to rest for 5 minutes. Serve with the fries.

STEAK WITH MUSHROOM AND RED WINE SAUCE

Choose your favourite cut of meat for this dish – keep it lean and organic, if possible, and always leave to rest before serving, to retain the tenderness of the steak.

SERVES 1
PREPARATION TIME 5 MINUTES, PLUS RESTING
COOKING TIME 12–15 MINUTES

1 tablespoon olive oil
2 shallots, diced
75 g (3 oz) chestnut mushrooms, sliced
100 ml (3½ fl oz) red wine
1 lean steak, about 175 g (6 oz)
crisp green salad, to serve

1 Heat the oil in a frying pan, add the shallots and cook for 3–4 minutes until softened. Add the mushrooms and cook for a further 4–5 minutes until tender. Pour in the wine, then bring to the boil and reduce by half.

2 Meanwhile, heat a griddle pan or preheat the grill until hot, then cook the steak to your liking. Leave to rest for 5 minutes.

3 Spoon the mushroom sauce over the steak and serve with a crisp green salad.

GRIDDLED CALVES' LIVER WITH SWEET POTATO MASH

Overcooked liver can be tough, so make sure the griddle pan is hot and cook the liver very quickly.

SERVES 4
PREPARATION TIME 15 MINUTES
COOKING TIME 30–35 MINUTES

1 teaspoon cumin seeds
3 tablespoons olive oil
2 large onions, sliced
2 thyme sprigs
500 g (1 lb) carrots, peeled and chopped
500 g (1 lb) sweet potatoes, peeled and chopped
400 g (13 oz) calves' liver, sliced
freshly ground black pepper

1 Heat a small, dry nonstick frying pan over a medium-low heat and dry-fry the cumin seeds for 2–3 minutes until golden brown and toasted. Set aside.

2 Heat 2 tablespoons of the oil in a separate frying pan, add the onions and thyme and cook over a low heat for about 30 minutes, stirring occasionally, until the onions start to caramelize.

3 Meanwhile, cook the carrots and sweet potatoes in a large saucepan of simmering water for 12–15 minutes until tender.

4 Towards the end of the cooking time, heat a griddle pan until hot and drizzle with the remaining oil. Cook the liver for 2–3 minutes on each side, depending on its thickness and until cooked to your liking.

5 Drain the carrots and potatoes, then return to the pan, add the toasted cumin seeds and mash together. Season the onions with pepper.

6 Serve the liver on the mash, topped with the onions.

MOROCCAN RACK OF LAMB

This is quite a spicy dish; if you want to make it milder just use less chilli powder. Be sure to ask your butcher to trim the excess fat off the rack of lamb.

SERVES 2
PREPARATION TIME 10 MINUTES,
PLUS RESTING
COOKING TIME 15–25 MINUTES

2 tablespoons olive oil
½ teaspoon ground cumin
½ teaspoon chilli powder
¼ teaspoon turmeric
¼ teaspoon paprika
¼ teaspoon ground coriander
2 garlic cloves, crushed
3 tablespoons chopped parsley
juice of ½ lemon
6-cutlet rack of lamb
steamed kale, to serve

1 Mix together the oil, all the spices, garlic, parsley and lemon juice in a bowl. Place the rack of lamb in a roasting tin and spread the spice mixture over the top.

2 Roast in a preheated oven, 200°C (400°F), Gas Mark 6, for 15–25 minutes, depending on how rare you like your lamb. Leave to rest for 5–6 minutes.

3 Serve with steamed kale.

LAMB AND ROSEMARY STEW

When cutting the lamb into cubes, try to trim off as much fat as you can to make this stew as healthy as possible.

SERVES 4
PREPARATION TIME 15 MINUTES
COOKING TIME 40 MINUTES

1 tablespoon olive oil
450 g (14½ oz) shoulder of lamb, cut into small cubes
1 onion, chopped
2 carrots, peeled and diced
2 garlic cloves, chopped
½ tablespoon chopped rosemary leaves
200 ml (7 fl oz) chicken stock
400 g (13 oz) can chopped tomatoes
grated rind and juice of 1 lemon
2 tablespoons chopped parsley

1 Heat the oil in a frying pan, add the meat, in batches if necessary, and cook until browned all over.

2 Add the onion and cook, stirring, for 3–4 minutes until starting to soften, then stir in the carrots, garlic and rosemary and cook for a further 3–4 minutes.

3 Pour in the stock and tomatoes and bring to the boil, then reduce the heat and simmer for 20 minutes.

4 Stir in the lemon rind and juice and chopped parsley and cook for a further minute before serving.

MUSHROOM AND SPINACH-STUFFED PORK TENDERLOIN

This impressive-looking dish is the perfect choice when you have friends coming to dinner.

SERVES 4
PREPARATION TIME 15 MINUTES, PLUS RESTING
COOKING TIME 55 MINUTES

1 tablespoon olive oil
2 back bacon rashers, chopped
½ small onion, diced
1 garlic clove, finely chopped
125 g (4 oz) chestnut mushrooms, chopped
½ tablespoon chopped thyme
½ tablespoon chopped rosemary
150 g (5 oz) baby spinach leaves
500–600 g (1–1¼ lb) pork tenderloin
steamed vegetables, to serve

1 Heat the oil in a frying pan, add the bacon and cook for 3–4 minutes until cooked through. Remove with a slotted spoon and set aside.

2 Add the onion and garlic to the pan and cook for 2–3 minutes until starting to soften. Add the mushrooms and herbs and cook for a further 3–4 minutes until the mushrooms are tender.

3 Stir in the spinach and toss until starting to wilt. Remove the pan from the heat and stir in the reserved bacon.

4 Cut down the middle of the tenderloin to open it like a book. Spread the stuffing mixture over the meat, then roll up to enclose the filling. Secure with cocktail sticks at the ends.

5 Place the stuffed tenderloin in a roasting tin and bake in a preheated oven, 190°C (375°F), Gas Mark 5, for 45 minutes until cooked through. Leave to rest for 10 minutes.

6 Slice the pork and serve with steamed vegetables.

BAKED PORK STEAKS WITH FENNEL AND BUTTERNUT SQUASH

A comforting and homely dish, this winter warmer can be cooked in one pot.

SERVES 4
PREPARATION TIME 15 MINUTES
COOKING TIME 45–50 MINUTES

2 tablespoons fennel seeds
1 tablespoon olive oil
4 pork loin steaks, fat trimmed
1 large onion, sliced
2 garlic cloves, sliced
500 g (1 lb) butternut squash, deseeded and cut into bite-sized pieces, skin on
2 fennel bulbs, trimmed and sliced
juice of 1 lemon
50 ml (2 fl oz) water

1 Crush the fennel seeds in a pestle and mortar and mix with half the oil. Rub the mixture over the pork chops and set aside.

2 Heat the remaining oil in a flameproof casserole or dish, add the onion and garlic and cook for 3–4 minutes until starting to soften, then add the squash and cook for a further 3–4 minutes.

3 Stir in the fennel, lemon juice and measurement water, cover with a lid and transfer to a preheated oven, 200°C (400°F), Gas Mark 6, for 25 minutes.

4 Remove the lid and stir gently, then place the pork chops on the top. Return to the oven, uncovered, and cook for a further 12–15 minutes until the pork is tender and cooked through.

PORK, APPLE AND SAGE BURGERS WITH HONEYED ONIONS

Everyone loves a burger and these are bursting with the flavour of fresh sage and apples.

SERVES 4
PREPARATION TIME 10 MINUTES, PLUS CHILLING
COOKING TIME 35 MINUTES

2 tablespoons olive oil
3 red onions, sliced
1 tablespoon clear honey
900 g (1¾ lb) minced pork
3 shallots, finely chopped
1 Bramley cooking apple, peeled and grated
1 egg, beaten
2 tablespoons chopped sage
freshly ground black pepper

1 Heat 1 tablespoon of the oil in a frying pan, add the onions and cook for 5 minutes until starting to soften, then drizzle with the honey and season with pepper. Reduce the heat to low and cook for 30 minutes, stirring occasionally.

2 Meanwhile, mix together the pork, shallots, apple, egg and sage in a large bowl, then shape into 4 burgers. Chill for 10 minutes.

3 Heat the remaining oil in a separate frying pan, add the burgers and cook for 5–6 minutes on each side, or until cooked through. Serve topped with the honeyed onions.

LEMON PORK AND MIXED PEPPER KEBABS

Ideal for the barbecue, these kebabs use lean pork tenderloin.

SERVES 4
PREPARATION TIME 15 MINUTES, PLUS MARINATING
COOKING TIME 12–15 MINUTES

2 tablespoons chopped rosemary
2 tablespoons olive oil
1 garlic clove, chopped
juice of 1 lemon
600 g (1¼ lb) pork tenderloin, cut into bite-sized pieces
2 red peppers, cored, deseeded and chopped
1 yellow pepper, cored, deseeded and chopped
freshly ground black pepper
lemon wedges, to serve

1 Mix together the rosemary, oil, garlic and lemon juice in a non-metallic bowl and season with pepper. Add the pork and mix to coat well. Leave to marinate for 15 minutes.

2 Thread the pork and mixed peppers alternately on to 8 metal skewers.

3 Cook on a barbecue or under a preheated hot grill for 12–15 minutes, turning and basting with the marinade occasionally, until the pork is cooked through and the peppers are tender. Serve with lemon wedges.

GRILLED PANCETTA-WRAPPED RADICCHIO

Grilling lettuce may sound strange, but it brings out the sweetness and gives it a tasty texture.

SERVES 4
PREPARATION TIME 5 MINUTES, PLUS STANDING
COOKING TIME 5–6 MINUTES

2 tablespoons olive oil
juice of ½ lemon
3 garlic cloves, crushed
1 tablespoon chopped rosemary
4 heads of radicchio, cut into quarters through the core end
8 slices of pancetta, halved lengthways
freshly ground black pepper

1 Whisk together the oil, lemon juice, garlic and rosemary in a large bowl and season with pepper. Add the radicchio and toss to coat, then leave to stand for 10 minutes.

2 Wrap each radicchio quarter in a halved slice of pancetta. Cook under a preheated hot grill or on a barbecue for 5–6 minutes, turning occasionally, until the edges are crisp and slightly charred. Serve drizzled with the remaining marinade.

SUMMER VEG AND EGGS WITH CRISPY BACON

You can use any variety of vegetables for this dish – even leftover veg work well.

SERVES 2
PREPARATION TIME 5 MINUTES
COOKING TIME 11–14 MINUTES

1 tablespoon olive oil
2 streaky bacon rashers, chopped
2 courgettes, roughly chopped
200 g (7 oz) cherry tomatoes, halved
50 g (2 oz) mangetout
3–4 basil leaves, roughly torn
2 large eggs

1 Heat the oil in a frying pan, add the bacon and cook until crisp. Remove from the pan with a slotted spoon and set aside.

2 Add the courgettes to the pan and cook for 5–6 minutes, stirring occasionally, until starting to soften. Add the tomatoes, mangetout and basil and cook for a further 1–2 minutes.

3 Make 2 hollows in the mixture and crack an egg into each hollow. Cover the pan with a lid or foil and cook for 2–3 minutes, or until the egg whites are set and the eggs are cooked to your liking. Serve sprinkled with the crispy bacon.

CHICKEN EN PAPILLOTE WITH ROASTED RATATOUILLE

Succulent chicken and roasted vegetables combine in this mouthwatering recipe.

SERVES 4
PREPARATION TIME 15 MINUTES
COOKING TIME 25–30 MINUTES

1 aubergine, cut into cubes
1 red pepper, cored, deseeded and chopped
1 yellow pepper, cored, deseeded and chopped
1 red onion, cut into wedges
2 courgettes, sliced
4 tablespoons olive oil
4 boneless, skinless chicken breasts, about 150 g (5 oz) each
8 tarragon sprigs
8 tablespoons water
freshly ground black pepper

1 Place the vegetables in a roasting tin and toss with 2 tablespoons of the oil. Roast in a preheated oven, 200°C (400°F), Gas Mark 6, for 25–30 minutes until just starting to char at the edges.

2 Meanwhile, place each chicken breast on a large piece of greaseproof paper. Add 2 sprigs of tarragon to each, then sprinkle each one with 2 tablespoons of the measurement water and season with pepper. Fold up the sides of the paper to seal the parcels and place on a baking sheet or in a roasting tin.

3 Cook the chicken in the oven alongside the vegetables for 15–18 minutes until cooked through.

4 Serve the chicken on a bed of the roasted vegetables.

CHICKEN TIKKA MASALA

This dish is made with a great homemade curry paste that can be stored in the refrigerator for 2 weeks and used for other recipes.

SERVES 4
PREPARATION TIME 15 MINUTES
COOKING TIME 45 MINUTES

1 tablespoon coconut oil
1 onion, chopped
1 red pepper, cored, deseeded and sliced
4 boneless, skinless chicken breasts, about 150 g (5 oz) each, cubed
400 g (13 oz) can chopped tomatoes
100 ml (3½ fl oz) water
2 tablespoons tomato purée
200 ml (7 fl oz) coconut milk
1 tablespoon chopped coriander, to garnish

FOR THE CURRY PASTE
2 cardamom pods
3 garlic cloves
2.5 cm (1 inch) piece of fresh root ginger, peeled and chopped
1 red chilli, deseeded
1 teaspoon ground cumin
1 teaspoon ground coriander
½ teaspoon turmeric
½ teaspoon garam masala

1 To make the curry paste, remove the seeds from the cardamom pods and place in a small food processor or blender with the remaining ingredients. Blend until smooth, adding a little water to loosen, if necessary. Transfer to an airtight container and store for up to 2 weeks in the refrigerator.

2 Heat the oil in a large frying pan, add the onion and cook over a low heat for 10–12 minutes until softened and lightly golden. Stir in the red pepper and 2 tablespoons of the curry paste and cook for a further 5 minutes.

3 Add the chicken, increase the heat and cook for 2 minutes until golden, then pour in the tomatoes and measurement water, add the tomato purée and bring to the boil. Reduce the heat, cover and simmer for 15 minutes, stirring occasionally, until the chicken is just cooked through.

4 Pour in the coconut milk and simmer for a further 10 minutes. Serve sprinkled with the chopped coriander.

CHICKEN AND BANANA KORMA

Adding bananas to a curry gives it a sweet, creamy texture.

SERVES 4
PREPARATION TIME 15 MINUTES
COOKING TIME 20–25 MINUTES

1 onion, chopped
2 garlic cloves, chopped
2 cm (¾ inch) piece of fresh root
    ginger, peeled and chopped
1 tablespoon olive oil
2 teaspoons mild curry powder
4 boneless, skinless chicken
    breasts, about 150 g (5 oz)
    each, cubed
50 g (2 oz) ground almonds
2 bananas, diced
400 ml (14 fl oz) chicken stock
2 tablespoons flaked almonds
3 tablespoons coconut milk
freshly ground black pepper
2 tablespoons chopped coriander,
    to garnish

1 Place the onion, garlic and ginger in a small food processor or blender and blend to a paste.

2 Place the paste and the oil in a large frying pan and cook over a medium heat for 2–3 minutes. Stir in the curry powder and cook for a further 3–4 minutes.

3 Add the chicken, ground almonds, bananas and stock and bring to the boil, then reduce the heat, cover and simmer for 10 minutes, or until the chicken is cooked through.

4 Meanwhile, heat a dry nonstick frying pan over a medium-low heat and dry-fry the flaked almonds for 2–3 minutes, shaking the pan occasionally, until golden brown and toasted. Set aside.

5 Stir the coconut milk into the curry and cook for a further 3–4 minutes, then season with pepper. Sprinkle with the chopped coriander and toasted almonds and serve.

CHICKEN AND CASHEW NUT CURRY

This rich curry could also be made with turkey if you prefer.

SERVES 4
PREPARATION TIME 15 MINUTES
COOKING TIME 25–35 MINUTES

60 g (2¼ oz) cashew nuts
2 teaspoons cumin seeds
1 tablespoon coriander seeds
½ teaspoon fennel seeds
2 curry leaves
2 tablespoons coconut oil
4 boneless, skinless chicken breasts, about 150 g (5 oz) each, cubed
1 onion, chopped
2 garlic cloves, crushed
2 cm (¾ inch) piece of fresh root ginger, grated
1 red chilli, deseeded and diced
500 ml (17 fl oz) chicken stock
75 g (3 oz) creamed coconut, chopped
450 g (14½ oz) spinach leaves
freshly ground black pepper
2 tablespoons chopped coriander, to garnish
steamed green vegetables, to serve (optional)

1 Heat a dry nonstick frying pan over a medium-low heat and dry-fry the cashews for 3–4 minutes, shaking the pan occasionally, until golden brown and toasted. Remove from the pan and set aside.

2 Add the seeds and curry leaves to the dry pan and dry-fry for 3–4 minutes until fragrant, then grind in a pestle and mortar or spice grinder.

3 Heat the oil in a large frying pan, add the chicken and cook for 3–4 minutes until browned. Add the onion, garlic, ginger and chilli and cook for a further 3–4 minutes, then stir in the ground spices and continue to cook for 2–3 minutes.

4 Pour in the stock, add the creamed coconut and bring to the boil, then reduce the heat and simmer for 10–15 minutes until the chicken is cooked through. Stir in the spinach and toasted cashew nuts and season with pepper.

5 Sprinkle with the chopped coriander and serve with steamed green vegetables, if liked.

CHICKEN CASSEROLE

∙∙

This easy family meal, made in one pot, is ideal for a cold winter's day.

∙∙

SERVES 4
PREPARATION TIME 10 MINUTES
COOKING TIME 1 HOUR 10 MINUTES

1 tablespoon olive oil
1 leek, trimmed, cleaned and chopped
1 celery stick, chopped
2 carrots, peeled and chopped
1 garlic clove, crushed
60 g (2¼ oz) mushrooms, halved
1 green pepper, cored, deseeded and chopped
1 tablespoon tomato purée
300 ml (½ pint) chicken stock
4 chicken thighs
4 chicken drumsticks
1 bay leaf
½ teaspoon dried marjoram
green vegetables, to serve

1 Heat the oil in a flameproof casserole, add the leek, celery, carrots and garlic and sauté for 4–5 minutes. Add the mushrooms and green pepper and cook for a further 4–5 minutes until softened.

2 Stir in the tomato purée, then pour in the stock. Add the chicken pieces, bay leaf and marjoram and bring to a simmer, then cover and cook for 1 hour, or until the chicken is tender and cooked through.

3 Serve the casserole with your choice of green vegetables.

SPICED WALNUT CHICKEN

This dish uses spices normally associated with sweet foods, but the flavours go particularly well with the chicken and walnuts.

SERVES 2
PREPARATION TIME 10 MINUTES
COOKING TIME 30–35 MINUTES

2 tablespoons olive oil
50 g (2 oz) walnuts, finely chopped
¼ teaspoon chilli powder
2 boneless, skinless chicken
   breasts, about 150 g (5 oz) each
1 shallot, diced
½ teaspoon ground cinnamon
½ teaspoon ground nutmeg
175 g (6 oz) grapes, halved
juice of ½ lemon
400 ml (14 fl oz) chicken stock

1 Mix together 1 tablespoon of the oil, the walnuts and chilli powder in a small bowl, then pat the mixture on to each chicken breast. Place the chicken on a baking sheet and bake in a preheated oven, 190°C (375°F), Gas Mark 5, for 30–35 minutes until the chicken is cooked through.

2 Meanwhile, heat the remaining oil in a frying pan, add the shallot and cook for 3–4 minutes until softened. Add the cinnamon and nutmeg and cook for a further 1–2 minutes.

3 Stir in the grapes, then pour in the lemon juice and stock and bring to a simmer. Cook for 6–8 minutes.

4 Serve the chicken with the sauce spooned over the top.

TURKEY MEATBALLS WITH COURGETTE TAGLIATELLE

Turkey is very lean, so is a good alternative to beef or lamb. Using thigh meat helps to keep these meatballs moist.

SERVES 4
PREPARATION TIME 15 MINUTES, PLUS COOLING AND CHILLING
COOKING TIME 20–25 MINUTES

1 tablespoon olive oil
1 red onion, diced
2 garlic cloves, finely chopped
1 teaspoon ground cumin
2 teaspoons ground coriander
400 g (13 oz) minced turkey
1 small bunch of coriander, finely chopped
400 g (13 oz) can chopped tomatoes
4 large courgettes
freshly ground black pepper

1 Heat half the oil in a frying pan, add the onion and cook for 4–5 minutes until softened. Add the garlic and spices and season with pepper, then cook for a further 1–2 minutes. Tip into a bowl and leave to cool for 5 minutes.

2 Add the turkey and chopped coriander to the cooled onions and combine well. Shape into 16 walnut-sized balls. Chill for 15 minutes.

3 Heat the remaining oil in a frying pan, add the turkey balls and cook for 3–4 minutes, turning occasionally, until browning.

4 Pour in the tomatoes, bring to a simmer and cook for a further 10–12 minutes until the meatballs are cooked through.

5 Meanwhile, cut the courgettes into thin strips using a vegetable peeler and cook in a saucepan of boiling water for 2–3 minutes, then drain.

6 Divide the courgette strips among 4 warmed bowls. Spoon over the turkey balls and serve.

DUCK WITH BROCCOLI AND ORANGE

Duck and orange is a classic combination.

SERVES 4
PREPARATION TIME 15 MINUTES, PLUS RESTING
COOKING TIME 20–25 MINUTES

4 duck breasts, about 150 g (5 oz) each
1 large head of broccoli, cut into florets
2 shallots, diced
1 red chilli, deseeded and finely diced
2 oranges, pith removed and segmented
freshly ground black pepper

1 Using a sharp knife, score the skin of the duck breasts in a criss-cross pattern. Season with pepper.

2 Heat an ovenproof frying pan until hot, add the duck, skin side down, and cook for 7–8 minutes until the fat runs out and the skin is golden. Turn the breasts over and cook for a further 1–2 minutes until browned. Remove 1–2 tablespoons of the duck fat and place in a separate frying pan.

3 Transfer the duck to a preheated oven, 200°C (400°F), Gas Mark 6, and cook for 8–10 minutes, depending on how rare you like your duck.

4 Meanwhile, put the broccoli in a steamer, cover and cook for 3–4 minutes until tender.

5 Remove the duck from the oven. Leave to rest for 5 minutes.

6 While the duck is resting, heat the reserved duck fat in the pan, add the shallots and chilli and cook for 3–4 minutes until softened. Add the steamed broccoli and toss to coat in the spicy oil, then sprinkle in the orange segments. Serve with the duck.

ROAST VENISON WITH WILD MUSHROOM SAUCE

This extravagant meal is perfect if you are entertaining dinner guests – they will never guess you are on a diet!

SERVES 4
PREPARATION TIME 10 MINUTES, PLUS RESTING
COOKING TIME 25–30 MINUTES

1 venison loin, about 600–650 g (1¼ lb)
2 teaspoons olive oil
1 tablespoon freshly ground black pepper
4 rosemary sprigs, leaves stripped and finely chopped
200 g (7 oz) wild mushrooms, cleaned
100 ml (3½ fl oz) beef stock
2 teaspoons Dijon mustard
steamed carrots and green beans, to serve

1 Using a sharp knife, lightly score the skin of the venison, then rub with the oil. Sprinkle the pepper and rosemary on to a chopping board, then rub the venison in the mixture to coat on all sides.

2 Heat a large frying pan until very hot, add the venison and cook for 2 minutes on each side, or until seared. Transfer to a roasting tin and place in a preheated oven, 200°C (400°F), Gas Mark 6, for 12–15 minutes, depending on how rare you like your meat. Leave to rest for 8–10 minutes.

3 Meanwhile, cook the mushrooms in the frying pan for 5–6 minutes until softened, then pour in the stock. Bring to the boil, then reduce the heat and simmer for 10 minutes, stirring in the mustard halfway through the cooking time.

4 Carve the venison into slices and spoon over the mushroom sauce. Serve with steamed carrots and green beans.

ROAST SQUASH WITH
WILD MUSHROOM SAUCE

6

VEGETARIAN

VEGETABLE KEBABS

These kebabs work well on a barbecue, and you can use any vegetables you like as long as they will stay on a skewer.

SERVES 4
PREPARATION TIME 10 MINUTES, PLUS SOAKING
COOKING TIME 10–12 MINUTES

2 tablespoons olive oil
2 tablespoons lemon juice
2 tablespoons chopped basil leaves
2 red peppers, cored, deseeded and chopped
1 yellow pepper, cored, deseeded and chopped
2 courgettes, cut into thick slices
1 large red onion, cut into wedges
freshly ground black pepper
bistro salad leaves, to serve

1 Soak 8 wooden skewers in water for at least 20 minutes to help prevent them from burning when cooking.

2 Mix together the oil, lemon juice and basil in a bowl and season with pepper. Place the vegetables in a large bowl, pour over the marinade and toss together.

3 Thread the vegetables on to the soaked skewers. Cook under a preheated medium grill or on a barbecue over a medium heat for 10–12 minutes, turning occasionally, until tender. Serve on bistro salad leaves.

GRIDDLED ASPARAGUS WITH POACHED EGG

This dish makes a satisfying lunch for one. You could also serve it as an impressive starter for a dinner party.

SERVES 1
PREPARATION TIME 5 MINUTES
COOKING TIME 5–7 MINUTES

10–12 asparagus spears, woody
   ends snapped off
1 egg
½ tablespoon olive oil
freshly ground black pepper

1 Blanch the asparagus in a saucepan of boiling water for 2 minutes. Drain, then refresh in a bowl of ice-cold water and drain again. Pat dry with kitchen paper.

2 Poach the egg in a small saucepan of simmering water for 3–5 minutes, or until cooked to your liking.

3 Meanwhile, sprinkle the oil over the asparagus and cook in a preheated hot griddle pan for 3–4 minutes until starting to char.

4 Place the asparagus on a warmed plate, top with the egg and season with pepper.

RATATOUILLE

A classic French dish, which is great served with grilled chicken or fish, or just on its own for vegetarians.

SERVES 4
PREPARATION TIME 15 MINUTES
COOKING TIME 35 MINUTES

4 large tomatoes
3 tablespoons olive oil
1 onion, sliced
3 garlic cloves, crushed
2 aubergines, chopped
3 courgettes, sliced
1 small bunch of basil, leaves only,
    roughly torn
freshly ground black pepper

1 Place the tomatoes in a heatproof bowl and pour over boiling water to cover. Leave for 1–2 minutes, then drain, cut a cross at the stem end of each tomato and peel off the skins. Halve and deseed, then set aside.

2 Heat the oil in a large frying pan, add the onion and garlic and cook for 3–4 minutes until starting to soften. Stir in the aubergines and courgettes and cook for a further 10 minutes, stirring occasionally.

3 Add the tomatoes and basil and season with pepper. Stir well, cover and cook for 20 minutes until the vegetables are tender.

ORIENTAL MARINATED VEGETABLES

Marinating is a wonderful way of infusing a dish with lots of different flavours. You can vary the vegetables according to the season, too.

SERVES 4
PREPARATION TIME 20 MINUTES, PLUS STANDING
COOKING TIME 3–4 MINUTES

2 tablespoons sesame seeds
75 g (3 oz) sugar snap peas
75 g (3 oz) baby corn
75 g (3 oz) broccoli, broken into florets
75 g (3 oz) carrots, peeled and cut into batons
4 spring onions, sliced
1 red pepper, cored, deseeded and cut into strips
50 g (2 oz) bean sprouts
1 small bunch of coriander, roughly chopped

FOR THE DRESSING
1 garlic clove
1 cm (½ inch) piece of fresh root ginger, peeled
2 tablespoons lemon juice
1 teaspoon sesame oil
2 tablespoons olive oil

1 Heat a dry nonstick frying pan over a medium-low heat and dry-fry the sesame seeds for 1–2 minutes, shaking the pan occasionally, until golden and toasted. Set aside.

2 Blanch the sugar snap peas, baby corn, broccoli and carrots in a large saucepan of boiling water for 2 minutes, then drain and refresh in a bowl of ice-cold water and drain again.

3 To make the dressing, place the garlic, ginger and lemon juice in a small food processor or blender and blend together. With the motor still running, add both the oils through the feeder tube until combined.

4 Place all the blanched and raw vegetables in a large serving bowl with the coriander. Add the dressing and toss together, then leave to stand for 5–10 minutes to allow the flavours to develop.

5 Serve sprinkled with the toasted sesame seeds.

VEGETABLE MASALA

Spice up your vegetables for a winter warming meal and, if you want even more heat, increase the amount of chilli powder in the dish.

2 garlic cloves
2.5 cm (1 inch) piece of fresh root
  ginger, peeled and chopped
400 g (13 oz) can chopped
  tomatoes
½ teaspoon cayenne pepper
2 tablespoons coconut oil
1 onion, chopped
1 red pepper, cored, deseeded
  and chopped
1 yellow pepper, cored, deseeded
  and chopped
2 carrots, peeled and chopped
2 parsnips, peeled and chopped
½ teaspoon garam masala
½ teaspoon chilli powder
1 small cauliflower, broken into
  florets
200 ml (7 fl oz) water
2 tablespoons flaked almonds,
  to garnish

1 Place the garlic and ginger in a small food processor or blender and blend together. Tip into a bowl, add the tomatoes and cayenne pepper and mix together.

2 Heat the oil in a large frying pan, add the onion and peppers and sauté for 8–10 minutes until softened.

3 Stir in the carrots, parsnips and spices and mix well, then cover and cook for 10 minutes, stirring the vegetables occasionally.

4 Add the cauliflower, tomato mixture and measurement water, bring to a simmer and cook for 20 minutes until all the vegetables are tender. Serve sprinkled with the flaked almonds.

7
SNACKS

BABA GANOUSH DIP WITH CRUDITÉS

This is a tasty, smoky dip that goes perfectly with crunchy veg as a quick snack.

SERVES 4
PREPARATION TIME 10 MINUTES, PLUS COOLING
COOKING TIME 35–40 MINUTES

1 large aubergine
1 garlic clove, crushed
1 tablespoon lemon juice
1 tablespoon tahini
½ tablespoon olive oil, plus extra if needed
½ teaspoon ground cumin
freshly ground black pepper
1 tablespoon chopped parsley, to garnish
vegetable sticks, such as carrots, peppers and celery, to serve

1 Place the aubergine directly on to an oven shelf in a preheated oven, 200°C (400°F), Gas Mark 6, and bake for 35–40 minutes until the skin has darkened all over. Alternatively, place the aubergine over an open flame on a gas hob or barbecue or under a very hot grill. Leave to cool.

2 When cool, peel off the aubergine skin and place the flesh in a food processor or blender. Add the remaining ingredients and blend until smooth. Season with pepper and add a little more oil if necessary.

3 Transfer the dip to a serving bowl and sprinkle with the parsley. Serve with the crudités for dipping.

CAULIFLOWER HUMMUS

Just because you can't have chickpeas, doesn't mean you can't have hummus!

SERVES 4
PREPARATION TIME 10 MINUTES, PLUS COOLING
COOKING TIME 25 MINUTES

1 cauliflower
2 teaspoons cumin seeds
5 tablespoons extra-virgin olive oil
1 garlic clove
1 tablespoon tahini
juice of 1 lemon
freshly ground black pepper

1 Break up the cauliflower into florets and cut the stalk into smaller chunks. Place in a roasting tin and toss with the cumin seeds and 1 tablespoon of the oil. Place in a preheated oven, 180°C (350°F), Gas Mark 4, for 25 minutes until tender. Leave to cool for 10 minutes.

2 Place the cooled cauliflower and garlic in a food processor and pulse until the mixture resembles breadcrumbs. Add the tahini and lemon juice and pulse again to mix. With the motor still running, slowly add the remaining oil through the feeder tube until it forms the consistency of hummus.

3 Season with pepper, transfer to a serving bowl and serve.

GUACAMOLE

A Mexican classic – you can add more chilli to make it hotter or blend it to make it smoother, whichever you prefer.

SERVES 2
PREPARATION TIME 10 MINUTES

1 large avocado
1 tomato, diced
juice of ½ lime
1 small bunch of coriander leaves
½ small red onion, finely diced
½ red chilli, deseeded and finely
    diced
vegetable crudités, to serve

1 Halve, stone and peel the avocado, then chop the flesh and place in a serving bowl.

2 Add the remaining ingredients and mash together with a fork to your preferred consistency.

3 Serve the guacamole with the vegetable crudités for dipping.

KALE CRISPS

These are a great alternative to potato crisps and far healthier. Make a large batch and serve as a snack before dinner.

SERVES 4
PREPARATION TIME 10 MINUTES
COOKING TIME 12 MINUTES

1 head of kale, chopped or torn
    into large pieces
1–2 tablespoons avocado oil
freshly ground black pepper or
    other seasoning (but not salt)

1 Line a baking sheet with nonstick baking paper.

2 Wash and thoroughly dry the kale leaves, then place in a large bowl and toss together with the oil.

3 Place the kale on the prepared baking sheet in a single layer and bake in a preheated oven, 180°C (350°F), Gas Mark 4, for 12 minutes.

4 Remove from the oven and immediately sprinkle with pepper or other seasoning. Leave to cool before serving.

SPICED NUTS AND SEEDS

These spicy nuts are handy for taking to work in a plastic pot, or even better served before dinner.

SERVES 6
PREPARATION TIME 5 MINUTES
COOKING TIME 13–16 MINUTES

1 tablespoon olive oil
juice of ½ lime
½ teaspoon chilli powder
½ teaspoon garam masala
½ teaspoon freshly ground black
  pepper
150 g (5 oz) mixed nuts and seeds,
  such as walnuts, almonds,
  pumpkin seeds and sunflower
  seeds
2 teaspoons clear honey

1 Line a baking sheet with nonstick baking paper.

2 Whisk together the oil and lime juice in a large bowl, then slowly add the spices and pepper, whisking to mix well.

3 Stir in the nuts and honey and mix well to thoroughly coat them with the spicy oil.

4 Spread the nuts on the prepared baking sheet and place in a preheated oven, 180°C (350°F), Gas Mark 4, for 5–6 minutes, then toss them slightly. Return to the oven and cook for a further 8–10 minutes until the nuts and seeds start to darken.

5 Leave to cool on the baking sheet before serving.

NUT AND SEED SAVOURY BISCUITS

These savoury biscuits are perfect for serving with Guacamole (see page 118). They will keep in an airtight container for up to 5 days.

MAKES 18–20
PREPARATION TIME 10 MINUTES
COOKING TIME 40–45 MINUTES

100 g (3½ oz) walnuts
100 g (3½ oz) blanched whole almonds
25 g (1 oz) ground flaxseeds
25 g (1 oz) poppy seeds
25 g (1 oz) desiccated coconut
75 g (3 oz) Savoy cabbage, roughly chopped
2 eggs
freshly ground black pepper

1 Line a large baking sheet with greaseproof paper.

2 Place the walnuts and almonds in a food processor and blitz until broken down into fine crumbs. Add the flaxseeds, poppy seeds, coconut and cabbage and process again until the mixture forms an even consistency. Season with pepper and add the eggs. Blend to a thick paste.

3 Spread the paste on to the paper on the prepared baking sheet. Top with another piece of greaseproof paper and roll out with a rolling pin until the paste is very thin. Remove the top sheet of paper and cut into 18–20 squares.

4 Bake in a preheated oven, 150°C (300°F), Gas Mark 2, for 40–45 minutes until golden. Transfer to a wire rack to cool.

SWEET POTATO WEDGES

These are delicious with one of the great dips in this book, such as Baba Ganoush (see page 116) or Cauliflower Hummus (see page 117).

SERVES 4
PREPARATION TIME 5 MINUTES
COOKING TIME 25–30 MINUTES

2 large sweet potatoes, cut into long wedges
2 tablespoons olive oil
1½ teaspoons smoked paprika
freshly ground black pepper

1 Toss the sweet potatoes with the oil, paprika and pepper in a large bowl, then tip into a roasting tin.

2 Place in a preheated oven, 200°C (400°F), Gas Mark 6, for 25–30 minutes until tender.

COURGETTE FRITTERS WITH POACHED EGGS

Fritters are quick and easy, and ideal for a packed lunch or picnic. You can replace the courgettes with sweetcorn or peas and mint.

SERVES 4
PREPARATION TIME 10 MINUTES
COOKING TIME 12–18 MINUTES

1 tablespoon olive oil
4 eggs
2 tablespoons chopped parsley,
    to garnish

FOR THE BATTER
200 g (7 oz) almond flour
1 egg, beaten
150 ml (¼ pint) non-dairy milk
200 g (7 oz) courgettes, diced
1 tablespoon chopped chives
freshly ground black pepper

1 To make the batter, place the flour in a large bowl and whisk in the egg and milk until smooth. Stir in the courgettes and chives and season with pepper.

2 Heat the oil in a frying pan, add tablespoons of the batter and cook for 2–3 minutes on each side until golden. Remove from the pan and keep warm. Repeat with the remaining batter until all the fritters are cooked.

3 Meanwhile, poach the eggs in a frying pan of simmering water for 3–5 minutes, or until cooked to your liking.

4 Divide the fritters among 4 warmed plates, top with the poached eggs and serve sprinkled with the parsley.

ROASTED PEPPERS

Roasted peppers are extremely versatile. You can fill them with vegetables, or roast them with garlic and leave them to cool, then slice and serve in a salad.

SERVES 4
PREPARATION TIME 10 MINUTES
COOKING TIME 25 MINUTES

2 red peppers, halved, cored and deseeded
2 yellow peppers, halved, cored and deseeded
1 red onion, cut into 8 wedges
18 cherry tomatoes
2 courgettes, halved and sliced
3 garlic cloves, sliced
2 tablespoons extra-virgin olive oil
1 teaspoon cumin seeds
2 tablespoons flaked almonds
freshly ground black pepper
crisp green salad, to serve

1 Place the pepper halves, cut side up, in a roasting tin and divide the remaining vegetables and garlic among them.

2 Sprinkle with the oil, cumin seeds and flaked almonds and season with pepper.

3 Roast in a preheated oven, 200°C (400°F), Gas Mark 6, for 25 minutes until tender. Serve with a crisp green salad.

SPICED CAULIFLOWER 'RICE'

As grains are not allowed on the Paleo diet, you may wish to try this 'rice' alternative to serve with curries or stir-fries.

SERVES 4
PREPARATION TIME 5 MINUTES
COOKING TIME 11–14 MINUTES

1 small cauliflower, broken into
  florets
1 tablespoon olive oil
1 onion, finely diced
½ teaspoon turmeric
½ teaspoon cumin seeds
150 ml (¼ pint) water

1 Place the cauliflower florets in a food processor and blitz until broken down into crumbs.

2 Heat the oil in a frying pan, add the onion and cook for 5–6 minutes until soft. Stir in the spices, then add the cauliflower and stir well to coat.

3 Pour in the measurement water, bring to a simmer and cook for 6–8 minutes until the cauliflower is tender.

LAMB KOFTAS

Easy to make and perfect for a summer barbecue, these lamb koftas can be made spicier by adding a diced red chilli.

SERVES 2
PREPARATION TIME 10 MINUTES
COOKING TIME 6–8 MINUTES

250 g (8 oz) minced lamb
½ teaspoon ground coriander
½ teaspoon ground cumin
1 garlic clove, crushed
½ tablespoon chopped mint
1 tablespoon olive oil
crisp green salad, to serve

1 Mix together the lamb, spices, garlic and mint in a bowl, then divide into 4 balls and shape into ovals. Thread the balls on to 2 metal skewers and brush with the oil.

2 Heat a griddle pan until very hot, add the koftas and cook for 3–4 minutes on each side until cooked through. Alternatively, cook the koftas on a barbecue. Serve with a crisp green salad.

HAM OMELETTE ROLL

This is a great recipe if you are hungry and want to eat on the go.

SERVES 1
PREPARATION TIME 2 MINUTES
COOKING TIME 4–6 MINUTES

1 tablespoon olive oil
3 eggs
pinch of chilli powder or paprika
1 slice of good-quality ham
1 spring onion, shredded

1 Heat the oil in a small frying pan. Beat together the eggs and chilli powder or paprika in a jug, then pour into the pan and cook for 3–4 minutes, moving the mixture around the pan, until the base is set. Flip the omelette over and cook for a further 1–2 minutes until cooked through.

2 Slide the omelette on to a plate, then place the ham on top and scatter over the spring onion. Roll up to enclose the ham and serve (or wrap in greaseproof paper to eat later).

PROSCIUTTO-WRAPPED MELON WEDGES

• •

This quick and easy snack could also be served as a starter for dinner.

• •

SERVES 4
PREPARATION TIME 8 MINUTES

1 gala melon
6 slices of prosciutto, halved
   lengthways

1 Halve, deseed and peel the melon, then cut into 12 wedges.

2 Wrap a thin slice of the prosciutto around each wedge of melon and serve – it really is that simple!

8

SWEET STUFF

BANANA AND RASPBERRY ICE CREAM

This ice cream is simple to make. The banana gives it a creamy texture and you can use your favourite fruit in place of the raspberries.

SERVES 2
PREPARATION TIME 15 MINUTES, PLUS FREEZING

1 banana, sliced
100 g (3½ oz) raspberries
100 ml (3½ fl oz) non-dairy milk

1 Place the banana slices and raspberries in a single layer on a baking sheet and freeze for at least 6 hours.

2 With the motor of a food processor running, slowly drop a few slices of banana, a few raspberries and a little of the milk into the bowl through the feeder tube. Keep adding each ingredient until the mixture forms a thick creamy ice cream. Serve immediately.

3 Alternatively, to freeze the ice cream, transfer the mixture to a freezer-proof container and place in the freezer for a few hours, then whisk the mixture with a fork to prevent ice crystals forming and making the ice cream too hard.

BANANA AND SUMMER BERRY SALAD

Summer berries and mint are a refreshing combination for a fruit salad.

SERVES 4
PREPARATION TIME 5 MINUTES, PLUS COOLING AND STANDING
COOKING TIME 1 MINUTE

juice of 1 orange
1 tablespoon clear honey
12–15 mint leaves, finely shredded
300 g (10 oz) strawberries, hulled and halved
250 g (8 oz) blueberries
225 g (7½ oz) raspberries
2 large bananas, sliced

1 Place the orange juice and honey in a small saucepan and heat together until the honey is just melted. Remove from the heat and leave to cool, then stir in the mint.

2 Place the berries and bananas in a large bowl and pour over the syrup. Leave to stand for 10 minutes before serving.

BLUEBERRY MOUSSE

A light, summery mousse, made creamier by the addition of omega-rich avocado.

SERVES 2
PREPARATION TIME 5 MINUTES, PLUS CHILLING

1 avocado
grated rind of 1 orange
150 g (5 oz) blueberries
1½ teaspoons clear honey
1 tablespoon ground almonds

1 Halve, stone and peel the avocado, then roughly chop the flesh and place in a food processor or blender with the remaining ingredients. Blend until smooth.

2 Divide between 2 glasses and chill until required.

BLUEBERRY AND ALMOND BAKEWELL SLICES

Ground almonds are great for making rich, tasty puddings and cakes. And, if you only have raspberries at hand, you can substitute them for the blueberries.

MAKES 9
PREPARATION TIME 10 MINUTES
COOKING TIME 22–25 MINUTES

75 g (3 oz) coconut oil, melted, plus extra for greasing
100 g (3½ oz) ground almonds
50 g (2 oz) coconut palm sugar
50 g (2 oz) coconut flour
40 g (1¾ oz) blueberries
3 eggs

1 Grease an 18 cm (7 inch) square cake tin and base-line with greaseproof paper.

2 Place the ground almonds, sugar, flour and blueberries in a bowl and lightly mix together.

3 Whisk together the melted oil and eggs in a jug, then stir into the dry ingredients. Spoon the mixture into the prepared tin and smooth the top.

4 Bake in a preheated oven, 180°C (350°F), Gas Mark 4, for 22–25 minutes until golden.

5 Cut into 9 squares, then remove from the tin and leave to cool on a wire rack.

WATERMELON AND STRAWBERRY SALAD

Watermelons and strawberries are best at the height of summer, when they are at their ripest.

SERVES 2
PREPARATION TIME 5 MINUTES,
** PLUS STANDING**

¼ watermelon, peeled and cut
  into chunks
125 g (4 oz) strawberries, hulled
  and halved
12 mint leaves, shredded
6 basil leaves, shredded
1 tablespoon clear honey

1 Mix together all the ingredients in a shallow non-metallic bowl, then leave to stand for 10 minutes before serving.

PEACHES AND BERRIES WITH LIME MINT SYRUP

A great summer dish when all the fruits are readily available.

SERVES 4
PREPARATION TIME 10 MINUTES, PLUS MARINATING

4 peaches, halved, stoned and sliced
60 g (2¼ oz) blueberries
juice of 1 lime
2 teaspoons clear honey
2 tablespoons chopped mint
100 g (3½ oz) raspberries
100 g (3½ oz) blackberries

1 Place the peaches, blueberries, lime juice, honey and mint in a non-metallic bowl and toss together. Cover and leave to marinate in the refrigerator for 1 hour.

2 Just before serving, toss in the raspberries and blackberries.

BAKED ALMOND AND GINGER PEACHES

Choose soft, ripe peaches for this sweet treat. You can also cook apricots or plums in the same way.

SERVES 4
PREPARATION TIME 10 MINUTES
COOKING TIME 20–22 MINUTES

2 knobs of stem ginger, diced
100 g (3½ oz) ground almonds
20 g (¾ oz) coconut oil
1 tablespoon clear honey
4 ripe peaches, halved and stoned

1 Mix together the ginger, ground almonds, oil and honey in a bowl.

2 Place the peaches, cut side up, in a roasting tin. Bake in a preheated oven, 200°C (400°F), Gas Mark 6, for 10 minutes, then remove from the oven and spoon in the almond filling. Return to the oven and bake for a further 10–12 minutes until golden and soft.

3 Serve the peaches drizzled with the pan juices.

GRILLED FRUIT BROCHETTES

These are such a fun way to eat fruit – and are perfect for a summer barbecue, too.

SERVES 4
PREPARATION TIME 20 MINUTES,
  PLUS STANDING
COOKING TIME 8–10 MINUTES

2 tablespoons clear honey
1 teaspoon green peppercorns
1 small bunch of mint
1 small bunch of basil
juice of 1 lime
200 ml (7 fl oz) water
1 mango, peeled and stoned
4 kiwi fruit, peeled
1 pineapple, peeled and cored
8 strawberries, hulled

1 Place the honey, peppercorns, half the herbs, lime juice and measurement water in a small saucepan, bring to the boil and boil for 1 minute. Remove from the heat and leave to stand for 15 minutes.

2 Meanwhile, cut all the fruit into bite-sized pieces and place in a non-metallic bowl.

3 Strain the syrup through a sieve over the fruit and leave to stand for at least 30 minutes (the longer you can leave it, the more intense the flavour will be).

4 Meanwhile, soak 12 small wooden skewers in water for at least 20 minutes to help prevent them from burning when cooking.

5 Thread the fruit on to the soaked skewers. Cook in a very hot griddle pan or on a barbecue, for 6–8 minutes, turning frequently, until slightly caramelized. Serve with a drizzle of the remaining marinade.

MANGO BAKED APPLES

Baked apples are usually filled with rich dried fruit; these are a little lighter, but still packed full of flavour.

SERVES 4
PREPARATION TIME 20 MINUTES,
**   PLUS STANDING**
COOKING TIME 15–20 MINUTES

1 mango, peeled, stoned and diced
grated rind and juice of 1 orange
75 g (3 oz) raisins
75 g (3 oz) walnuts, chopped
½ teaspoon ground cinnamon
4 dessert apples

1 Place the mango and orange rind and juice in a bowl. Add the raisins and leave to stand for 15 minutes. Stir in the walnuts and cinnamon.

2 Core and peel the apples, then place in a shallow ovenproof dish and spoon the mango mixture into the centre of each one, pressing it down well. Pile any remaining mixture on top.

3 Bake in a preheated oven, 180°C (350°F), Gas Mark 4, for 15–20 minutes, basting once, until the apples are softened and there is plenty of juice. Serve with the juice from the pan drizzled over the top.

MANGO 'CHEESECAKES'

This recipe for 'cheesecake' is a very good substitute for the real thing.

SERVES 4
PREPARATION TIME 15 MINUTES,
PLUS COOLING AND CHILLING
COOKING TIME 10 MINUTES

50 g (2 oz) ground almonds
25 g (1 oz) hazelnut butter
25 g (1 oz) coconut palm sugar
1 tablespoon desiccated coconut
1 avocado
2 mangoes, peeled, stoned and
    chopped
grated rind of 1 orange

1 Place the ground almonds and hazelnut butter in a bowl and mix together using the back of a spoon until the mixture resembles coarse breadcrumbs. Stir in the sugar.

2 Spoon the mixture into 4 ramekins and press down evenly. Bake in a preheated oven, 200°C (400°F), Gas Mark 6, for 10 minutes. Leave to cool.

3 Meanwhile, heat a dry nonstick frying pan over a medium-low heat and dry-fry the desiccated coconut, shaking the pan occasionally, until golden brown and toasted. Set aside.

4 Halve, stone and peel the avocado, then chop the flesh and place in a food processor or blender with the mangoes and orange rind. Blend until smooth.

5 Divide the mixture among the ramekins, then sprinkle with the toasted coconut. Chill for 15 minutes before serving.

SPICY GRIDDLED PINEAPPLE

Pineapple is perfect for cooking in a griddle pan as it starts to caramelize quickly. Chilli goes well with this robust fruit, or you could try black pepper as an alternative.

SERVES 4
PREPARATION TIME 5 MINUTES
COOKING TIME 13–15 MINUTES

8 slices of fresh pineapple, skin removed
3 teaspoons clear honey
pinch of chilli flakes
pinch of ground cinnamon

1 Heat a griddle pan or frying pan until very hot, add the pineapple and cook for 6–7 minutes on each side until starting to caramelize.

2 Add the remaining ingredients and cook until the mixture starts to bubble – this will not take long.

3 Serve the pineapple slices drizzled with the spicy honey.

CARAMELIZED FIGS WITH CASHEW CREAM

Figs don't need much doing to them to make them any more delicious, but this recipe brings out their sweetness.

SERVES 2
PREPARATION TIME 5 MINUTES
COOKING TIME 2–4 MINUTES

2 figs
2 teaspoons coconut oil
60 g (2¼ oz) cashew nuts
75 ml (3 fl oz) non-dairy milk
ground cinnamon, for sprinkling

1 Cut the stems off the figs, then cut in half widthways.

2 Melt the oil in a hot griddle pan, add the figs, cut side down, and cook for 1–2 minutes on each side, or until starting to caramelize

3 Meanwhile, place the cashews in a food processor and blitz until finely ground. With the motor still running, slowly add the milk through the feeder tube until it forms a creamy consistency

4 Remove the figs from the pan, sprinkle with cinnamon and serve with the cashew cream.

APPLE, ALMOND AND CINNAMON MUFFINS

These muffins are super rich. You can also vary the recipe by adding your favourite flavours to the basic mix.

MAKES 6
PREPARATION TIME 10 MINUTES
COOKING TIME 28–30 MINUTES

125 g (4 oz) ground almonds
125 g (4 oz) coconut palm sugar
1 dessert apple, cored, peeled
  and diced
½ teaspoon ground cinnamon
125 g (4 oz) coconut oil, melted
3 eggs, beaten

1 Mix together the ground almonds, sugar, apple and cinnamon in a bowl.

2 Whisk together the melted oil and eggs in a jug, then pour into the dry ingredients and mix together well. Spoon the mixture into 6 holes of a muffin tin.

3 Bake in a preheated oven, 180°C (350°F), Gas Mark 4, for 28–30 minutes until risen and golden. Remove from the tin and leave to cool on a wire rack.

PEAR AND ORANGE CRUMBLE WITH ALMOND CREAM

Just because you can't have dairy, doesn't mean you can't have cream. Here, nuts and non-dairy milk make an excellent cream equivalent.

SERVES 4
PREPARATION TIME 15 MINUTES
COOKING TIME 20 MINUTES

4 pears, cored and sliced
1 orange
75 g (3 oz) ground almonds
25 g (1 oz) coconut oil
pinch of ground nutmeg
2 teaspoons clear honey
125 g (4 oz) blanched almonds
150 ml (¼ pint) non-dairy milk

1 Place the pears in a shallow ovenproof dish. Grate the rind of the orange into a separate bowl.

2 Using a sharp knife, remove the peel and pith from the orange. Holding the orange over the pears to catch the juice, cut out the segments and add to the pears.

3 Stir the ground almonds into the orange rind, then rub in the coconut oil, using the back of a spoon, until it resembles coarse breadcrumbs. Stir in the nutmeg.

4 Sprinkle the crumble over the pears and drizzle with the honey. Bake in a preheated oven, 200°C (400°F) Gas Mark 6, for 20 minutes.

5 Meanwhile, place the blanched almonds in a food processor and blitz until finely ground. With the motor still running, gradually add the milk through the feeder tube until it forms a creamy consistency.

6 Serve the crumble warm, with the almond cream.

HONEYED TANGERINES

A slight change from caramelized oranges, tangerines have a flavour that is unique, and this recipe brings out the best in them.

SERVES 2
PREPARATION TIME 5 MINUTES
COOKING TIME 10–12 MINUTES

3 tangerines
2 tablespoons clear honey
1 cinnamon stick
100 ml (3½ fl oz) water

1 Peel and thinly slice the tangerines, then divide the slices between 2 plates.

2 Place the honey, cinnamon stick and measurement water in a small saucepan and heat over a medium heat, then simmer gently until the syrup turns golden and thickens slightly.

3 Pour the caramel over the tangerine slices and serve.

9

DRINKS

BREAKFAST SMOOTHIE

You can make a smoothie from pretty much any fruit and even some vegetables, so experiment with your favourite flavours.

SERVES 1
PREPARATION TIME 5 MINUTES

150 g (5 oz) fresh or frozen mixed berries
1 small ripe banana, chopped
1 tablespoon flaked almonds
100 ml (3½ fl oz) water
1 teaspoon clear honey (optional)

1 Place the berries, banana, flaked almonds and measurement water in a blender and blend until smooth. Add a little more water to loosen the consistency, if necessary.

2 Add honey to taste, if liked, and pour into a glass. Serve immediately.

GREEN SMOOTHIE

This smoothie is a real health boost – add any greens you love and think of it as a summer savoury drink.

SERVES 1
PREPARATION TIME 5 MINUTES

1 apple
1 celery stick
¼ cucumber, chopped
½ teaspoon grated fresh root
    ginger
small handful of parsley leaves
1 small garlic clove
juice of ½ lemon
300 ml (½ pint) mineral water
freshly ground black pepper
ice cubes, to serve

1 Place all the ingredients in a blender and season with pepper, then blend until smooth.

2 Pour over ice cubes in a glass and serve immediately.

RASPBERRY AND APPLE SMOOTHIE

Adding ground almonds to this smoothie gives it a rich, creamy consistency. Use any non-dairy milk you like; there are now lots to choose from.

SERVES 1
PREPARATION TIME 5 MINUTES

20 g (¾ oz) ground almonds
60 g (2¼ oz) raspberries
1 dessert apple, chopped
300 ml (½ pint) non-dairy milk

1 Place all the ingredients in a blender and blend until smooth.

2 Pour the smoothie into a glass and serve immediately.

CREAMY COOL CUCUMBER SMOOTHIE

This green smoothie is full of goodness and tastes really fresh. You can also add any of your favourite herbs or a pinch of chilli for a little extra punch.

SERVES 2
PREPARATION TIME 5 MINUTES

1 avocado
juice of ½ lime
⅓ cucumber, chopped
pinch of freshly ground black
    pepper
ice cubes, to serve

1 Halve, stone and peel the avocado, then roughly chop the flesh and place in a blender with the remaining ingredients. Blend with enough water to form a creamy, drinkable consistency.

2 Pour over ice cubes in 2 glasses and serve immediately.

APPLE AND GINGER JUICE

You will need a juicing machine to create this drink. Making your own juice is a great way of getting lots of healthy nutrients into your body. Don't overdo the fruit though, as this will add sugar to your diet.

SERVES 1
PREPARATION TIME 3 MINUTES

2 dessert apples
2 carrots
1 cm (½ inch) piece of fresh
    root ginger
½ lemon

1 Place all the ingredients in a juicer and process.

2 Pour into a glass and serve immediately.

SPICED ALMOND MILK

If you like drinking ice-cold milk, this is the non-dairy equivalent, with a touch of spice. It takes a little time to prepare, but you can make a large batch and store it in the refrigerator.

SERVES 2
PREPARATION TIME 15 MINUTES, PLUS SOAKING

175 g (6 oz) raw almonds
850 ml (1½ pints) mineral or filtered water
pinch of ground cinnamon
ice cubes, to serve

1 Place the almonds in a bowl and cover with water. Leave to soak in the refrigerator for 24 hours.

2 Drain the almonds, then place in a blender with the measurement water and blend until the nuts are completely broken down.

3 Put a couple of layers of muslin in a sieve, then strain the milk into a jug, squeezing out the excess moisture from the almonds.

4 Pour over ice cubes in 2 glasses, sprinkle with cinnamon and serve immediately.

ICED MINT TEA

Green tea is rich in antioxidants and has been shown to have many health benefits. Make a jug of this refreshing iced tea for those days when you need a thirst quencher.

SERVES 4–6
PREPARATION TIME 2 MINUTES,
**   PLUS COOLING AND CHILLING**

handful of mint leaves
3–4 green tea bags
1 litre (1¾ pints) boiling water
clear honey (optional)
ice cubes, to serve

1 Gently bruise half the mint leaves and place them in a large heatproof jug.

2 Add the tea bags and pour over the measurement water. Cover and leave to cool, then chill for 3–4 hours.

3 Remove the tea bags and mint, then stir in the remaining mint leaves and a little honey, if liked.

4 Pour over ice cubes in glasses and serve immediately.

MANGO AND FLAXSEED SMOOTHIE

Ground flaxseeds are a great source of omega-3 essential fats, and also help to support the detoxification process, which is very important if you are trying to lose weight.

SERVES 1
PREPARATION TIME 5 MINUTES

1 ripe mango, peeled, stoned and chopped
150 ml (¼ pint) non-dairy milk
2 teaspoons ground flaxseeds
½ teaspoon clear honey (optional)
ice cubes, to serve

1 Place the mango, milk and flaxseeds in a blender and blend until smooth. Add the honey to taste, if liked.

2 Pour over ice cubes in a glass and serve immediately.

INDEX